How the COVID-19 Pandemic Is Affecting Your Health and Your Healthcare

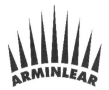

How the COVID-19 Pandemic is Affecting Your Health and Your Healthcare

Don L Goldenberg, MD

Emeritus Professor of Medicine, Tufts University School of Medicine

Adjunct Faculty, Departments of Medicine and Nursing

Oregon Health Sciences University

Armin Lear Press
825 Wildlife
Estes Park, CO 80517

To the countless patients and their heroic healthcare workers
who have endured during this pandemic

ACKNOWLEDGEMENTS

To my wife, Patty, always by my side, and my two amazing daughters and our grandchildren. Thanks to Howard Ory for his counsel and to Maryann Karinch, who helped prepare and publish this book in a timely fashion.

CONTENTS

INTRODUCTION

  Am I infected?

  How to get tested?

  Impact on Non-COVID patients with urgent medical conditions

  Age and co-morbidity

  Extended care facilities

  Health care workers

  Obesity and diabetes

  Immunosuppression

  Primary Care Offices

  Telemedicine

  Business as Usual?

  In-patients Recovering from Acute COVID-19 Infection

  In the Rest of Us

  Information: Tuning In and Tuning Out

  Coping, Lifestyle

  Exercise

  Sleep

CONCLUDING REMARKS

Introduction

The COVID-19 pandemic is the most significant medical event of our generation. In just two months, it became the leading cause of death per day in the United States, surpassing heart disease and cancer. COVID-19 has directly or indirectly impacted everyone's personal health and forever changed healthcare delivery in the United States. This book will bring you up to date with the most significant changes that have affected us during the initial phase of the pandemic.

"Up to date" is an assertion we can make because our publisher is committed to bringing out a new version of this book whenever a significant shift occurs in our knowledge of virus detection, prevention, and treatments.

We will begin with a review of what we know about acute COVID-19 infection: What are the signs and symptoms of acute infection and how to get tested? Then we will discuss the impact of the pandemic on urgent non-COVID related medical conditions, such as heart attacks and stroke.

Next, the general risk factors for COVID infection, including age and co-morbidities, most notably diabetes, obesity and immunosuppression, are discussed. The increased risk for nursing home residents and for health care workers will be examined.

Then, we will review the transformations in healthcare practice as a result of the pandemic. This has been especially important in primary care, with widespread incorporation of telemedicine. Practice-related changes, including integrated teams and reimbursement strategies are detailed.

Next, we will consider the mental health fallout, first for patients infected with COVID-19 and then for the general population. The final section discusses self-management. How do we get the most reliable medical information and when do we need to tune out? What are recommended lifestyle and coping strategies? The important role of exercise and sleep is reviewed.

The first forty years of my career were spent primarily taking care of patients with rheumatic and immunologic diseases. Administrative duties included supervising an internal medicine residency program and developing the first primary care training program at Boston City Hospital. My early research included studies on the role of infections in arthritis and related disorders. During the past 30 years, much of my research was dedicated to chronic pain disorders, most particularly fibromyalgia. I was Professor of Medicine at Boston University School of Medicine and Tufts University School of Medicine. I have been the author of over 200 peer-reviewed medical articles, and interviewed for the media, including on *The Today Show*, *Good Morning America, The New York Times, The Boston Globe* and *The New Yorker.* Honors have included the Marion Ropes Lifetime Achievement Award from the Massachusetts Arthritis Foundation, named a Master, American

College of Rheumatology, 2009 and selected for *Best Doctors in America*, Woodward & White, 2010-2016.

After retiring from practice five years ago and moving to Portland, Oregon, I have continued to stay involved in clinical research and teaching in my role as Emeritus Professor of Medicine at Tufts University School of Medicine and adjunct faculty member in the Departments of Medicine and Nursing at Oregon Health Sciences University. During the past few months I have authored a number of medical journal articles, published in *Practical Pain Management*, on the impact of COVID-19 in the rheumatic diseases, diabetes and other immune diseases. I am the Section Editor for the *UptoDate* topic, Coronavirus disease 2019 (COVID-19): Care of patients with systemic rheumatic disease during the pandemic.

Since the pandemic began, and following shelter-in-place guidelines, I have spent the better part of each day combing the literature on the effect of the pandemic on aspects of health care most important to the public. This has included daily reviews of every article listed in PubMed on COVID-19 or related coronavirus headings. During the months of February through May, 2020, this has included more than 4500 peer-reviewed papers on COVID-19 related topics. I have also searched media sources, focusing on pertinent articles from the *New York Times, The Boston Globe, The Washington Post* and STAT News. I have collected and collated what I consider to be the most essential information to serve as the backbone of this book.

Since the focus is to examine the effect of this pandemic on the public and their general healthcare, I did not include any medical information on basic science or epidemiology of COVID-19. I have chosen to stay away from predictions and speculate as to what comes next. This is why I have not included any discussion of potential therapies and vaccines. What is said today may not be accurate in the near future.

We have all been deluged with an avalanche of media news on the pandemic. This book is an attempt to synthesize current information, providing an overview and general perspective on how COVID-19 has affected each of us. This review is not intended to deliver proscriptive medical information and that only should be accessed from your personal healthcare providers.

1
The Acute Infection

Am I Infected?

During the first week of March my 50-year-old daughter had daily fever, up to 102°F, a hacking cough, total body aches and exhaustion. She became progressively short of breath. Her primary care doctor was not seeing patients and told her to stay home and self-isolate, which she did. Around the third day of spiking fevers, she noticed that her sense of smell and taste were off. Racked with exhaustion, fever and trouble breathing, she went to an urgent care center. Her lungs did not sound congested and the doctor thought that she did not have pneumonia. A flu test was negative. She was given an antibiotic but told that she may have COVID infection. At the time, there was no readily available coronavirus testing. After three more days of unrelenting fever and cough, my daughter's PCP suggested that she go to the hospital emergency room (ER). Fortunately, her fever broke the next day before she was forced to make the dreaded trip to the ER.. Her scenario followed the script described by Dr. Harlan Krumholz in *The New York Times* on April 1, 2020, "They test you for influenza by sticking a swab far up your nose, and you are told the test came back negative, you don't have flu. They tell you they are saving the Covid-19 tests for those who are even worse off than you are. You go home with a prescription for antibiotics, possibly because they don't know what else to do, and you read about celebrities who are testing positive but don't seem so sick."[1]

My daughter's symptoms were typical of acute COVID-19 infection[2]. Classic symptoms, recently updated by the Centers for Disease Control, include:

- Fever, usually greater than 38°C
- Dry, hacking cough
- Shortness of breath
- Chills with shaking
- Muscle aches and pain
- Headache
- Loss of taste and smell
- Sore throat

Some caveats to remember: The vast majority of patients have mild symptoms, and this doesn't include people who never get symptoms despite confirmed evidence of infection. In some people COVID seems like a bit of a cold and goes away in a few days. The symptoms may appear from two days to two weeks after exposure. Up to 50 percent of patients do not have fever

---

[1] Harlan M. Krumholz. If you have coronavirus symptoms, assume you have the illness, even if you test negative. *The New York Times*. April 1, 2020.

[2] CDC website. Coronavirus Disease 2019. Symptoms of Coronavirus. Accessed 5/6/2020.

initially. Ten to twenty percent of patients have nausea, vomiting or diarrhea. However, diarrhea may be more common than initially recognized and a recent report found that nearly 50 percent of COVID-19 patients reported diarrhea[3]. In contrast to typical influenza, most COVID patients do not experience a runny nose or nasal congestion. The loss of taste and smell is unusual in any other acute infection and has been present in 50-80 percent of COVID cases.[4]

During the first few months, almost all infection screening was done by telephone. A number of standardized telephone triage scripts for healthcare personnel have been published, including by Kay, *et al* in the *New England Journal of Medicine* which asks three questions:

1. Do you have a fever, chills, new or worsening cough, shortness of breath, sore throat, myalgias, gastrointestinal symptoms or other flu-like symptoms?

2. Have you traveled to any country or regions with positive cases of COVID-19 in the last 14 days?

3. Have you been in close contact with anyone, including health care workers, confirmed to have COVID-19?

Patients who screen positive for possible COVID should then be further evaluated, which can be done in-person or remotely. The status of any

---

[3] Klopfenstein T, et al. Diarrhea: An underestimated symptom in Coronavirus disease 2019. *Clin Res Hepatol Gastroenterol.* 2020 Apr 27.
[4] Beltrán-Corbellini Á, et al. Acute-onset smell and taste disorders in the context of Covid-19: a pilot multicenter PCR-based case-control study. *Eur J Neurol.* 2020 Apr 22. doi: 10.1111/ene.14273

respiratory symptoms must be carefully assessed. Greenhalgh and colleagues suggested targeted queries for healthcare providers to ask:

- "Are you so breathless that you are unable to speak more than a few words?"
- "Are you breathing harder or faster than usual when doing nothing at all?"
- "Are you so ill that you've stopped doing all of your usual daily activities?"

Any person with a temperature above 38°C, respiratory rate above 20 breaths/minute, and heart rate above 100 beats/minute should be seen in an Emergency Room or admitted to hospital, preferably in a setting dedicated to COVID patients. Mental confusion and low urinary output are particularly ominous signs.

Many clinics and hospitals have established dedicated units for the evaluation of patients with suspected COVID-19 infection and active respiratory symptoms. The University of California, San Francisco (UCSF) Health system has utilized a "respiratory clinic".[5] Any patient with cough, fever, shortness of breath or similar acute pulmonary symptoms receives an examination and testing in that dedicated respiratory clinic. The unit performs pulse oximetry, portable chest X-ray and blood tests, tests for acute infection and keeps the patient isolated from other patients, clinic or hospital staff.

---

[5] Harmes K, et al. Implementation of Primary Care Pandemic Plan: Respiratory Clinic Model Posted on *Annals of Family Medicine* COVID-19. Collection 2020.

In some patients the shortness of breath emerges late, such as a week after other symptoms, and it may get severe without much warning. Initially many patients report very little breathing problems despite evidence of low oxygen saturation with pulse oximetry or evidence of acute pneumonia on Chest X-ray. Dr. Richard Levitan described COVID-19 patients that he was taking care of at Bellevue Hospital in New York, "But when Covid pneumonia first strikes, patients don't feel short of breath, even as their oxygen levels fall. And by the time they do, they have alarmingly low oxygen levels and moderate-to-severe pneumonia (as seen on chest X-rays). Normal oxygen saturation for most persons at sea level is 94 to 100 percent; Covid pneumonia patients I saw had oxygen saturations as low as 50 percent. To my amazement, most patients I saw said they had been sick for a week or so with fever, cough, upset stomach and fatigue, but they only became short of breath the day they came to the hospital. Their pneumonia had clearly been going on for days, but by the time they felt they had to go to the hospital, they were often already in critical condition. From a public health perspective, we've been wrong to tell people to come back only if they have severe shortness of breath. Toughing it out is not a great strategy."[6]

Dr. Levitan recommended that we all have pulse oximeters at home and use them as we would a thermometer to check for fever, "Pulse oximetry is no more complicated than using a thermometer. These small devices turn on with one button and are placed on a fingertip. In a few seconds, two numbers

---

[6] Richard Levitan. The Infection That's Silently Killing Coronavirus Patients. *The New York Times*. April 20, 2020.

are displayed: oxygen saturation and pulse rate. Pulse oximeters are extremely reliable in detecting oxygenation problems and elevated heart rates. "[7] I ordered a pulse oximeter online six weeks ago. I still haven't received it.

Dr. Ilan Schwartz, an infectious disease specialist at the University of Alberta described a "a very nasty second wave…After the initial symptoms, things plateau and maybe even improve a little bit, and then there is a secondary worsening."[8] Dr Leora Horwitz, professor of population health and medicine at New York University Langone Health stated, "With any other disease, most people, after a week of symptoms, they're like 'OK, things will get better'. With Covid, I tell people that around a week is when I want you to really pay attention to how you're feeling. Don't get complacent and feel like it's all over."[9]

If you can't get a pulse oximeter, some experts have suggested using a simple self-test called the Roth score.[10] You take a deep breath and start counting to yourself as fast as you can, while holding your breath. The Roth score is calculated as the duration of time you held your breath and the highest number you counted. If you can't get to number 10 without another breath, your oxygen saturation has likely fallen below 90 and you need to be evaluated by a healthcare professional quickly.

---

[7] *Ibid*
[8] Tara Parker-Pope. Why Days 5 to 10 Are So Important When You Have Coronavirus. *The New York Times*. April 30, 2020.
[9] *Ibid*
[10] Chorin E, et al. Assessment of respiratory distress by the Roth Score. *Clin Cardiol*. 2016;39:636.

Patients with COVID reported their symptoms to the *New York Times* in quite striking fashion,[11] "And the heavy, hoarse cough, my God. The cough rattled through my whole body. You know how a car sounds when the engine is sputtering? That is what it sounded like." Another patient described the chest pain, "On Day 10, I woke up at 2:30 a.m. holding a pillow on my chest. I felt like there was an anvil sitting on my chest. Not a pain, not any kind of jabbing—just very heavy." One patient described the intertwined chest pain and shortness of breath just as my daughter had told me, "Doing anything other than laying (sic) in bed and sleeping was difficult. You had to be in the right position in order for your chest to not hurt. Or you had to be in a certain position in order to be able to take a full, comfortable breath. It's like deep inside your chest. You feel it. Something is definitely inside of me, and I'm definitely infected with something."[12]

As the pandemic rolls on, more unusual manifestations of COVID infection have been seen. Some involve multi-systemic symptoms suggestive of an inflammatory/immune disease. Skin manifestations may include localized or more generalized rashes or skin lesions, often seen by rheumatologists with systemic vasculitis. These include painful skin lesions usually in the feet, dubbed as COVID-toe, but also in the fingers[13]. Akin to what dermatologists describe as chilblains, Dr. Lindy Fox, a dermatologist in San Francisco, said,

---

[11] Antonio de Luca. 'An Anvil Sitting on My Chest': What It's Like to Have Covid-19. *The New York Times*. May 6, 2020.

[12] *Ibid*

[13] Roni Caryn Rabin. What is Covid Toe? Maybe a Strange Sign of Coronavirus Infection. *New York Times*. May 1, 2020.

"All of a sudden, we are inundated with toes, I've got clinics filled with people coming in with new toe lesions. And it's not people who had chilblains before — they've never had anything like this."

Children with COVID-19 have developed rashes, especially of the back and face, eye inflammation, abdominal pain as well as kidney and heart abnormalities, a new illness termed multisystem inflammatory syndrome.[14] The picture is similar to a rare immune disease, Kawasaki disease. Kawasaki disease is most common in children from East Asia who typically present with acute fever, rash, lymph node swelling and may develop cardiac complications, including heart inflammation or even heart failure. Coronary artery aneurysms, small dilated blood vessels, are telltale and dangerous. In the cases related to COVID-19, coronary aneurysms have not been described but rather the cardiac picture is one of diffuse inflammation, a myocarditis. The cause of Kawasaki disease is unknown but, as is the case for many systemic, inflammatory diseases, it has been hypothesized that an infection, such as a virus, triggers an immune response, leading to widespread inflammation. Kawasaki disease does occur in epidemics with evidence for geographic transmission[15]. It usually is self-limited, running a two-week course.

On May 4, 2020 the New York City Health Department issued a bulletin describing 15 cases of multisystem, inflammatory disease in children and the next day the New York Times suggested that at least fifty children had been

---

[14] Joseph Goldstein, Pan Belluck. Children are falling ill with a baffling ailment related to Covid-19. *New York Times*. May 5, 2020.

[15] Yanagawa H, et al. A nationwide incidence survey of Kawaski disease in 1985-1986 in Japan. *J Infect Dis* 1988;158:1296.

hospitalized with the syndrome[16]. More children throughout the country are now reported daily. The timing in relation to COVID infection suggests that this is an inflammatory/immune response. Therapy with corticosteroids or immunoglobulin, similar to that used in Kawasaki disease or any systemic vasculitis, has been generally effective.

Testing for COVID-19

Testing for COVID-19 is the only way to know for certain if a person is infected. Once that is known, clinicians can decide the next course of action: should a person self-isolate, seek medical care in-person or immediately be hospitalized. These decisions are made based on severity of symptoms.

As the novel virus swept across the world in record fashion, there was a critical lag time before diagnostic tests were developed and made available. Therefore, during the first few months of the pandemic, testing for COVID-19 infection was limited primarily to high risk patients who had symptoms of the infection, patients in long-term care facilities or patients over 65 years of age.

Unfortunately, many people went untested. Even by late April, less than 50 percent of primary care providers (PCP) had adequate testing capacity, including one-third of PCPs who reported no testing capability. One PCP complained, "It is appalling to me that we don't have broader testing capabilities. I had a patient two days ago who absolutely should have been tested. But because she hadn't traveled internationally, or had a known contact

---

[16] Goldstein, 2020.

with COVID, we couldn't. She was flu negative. It's insane. We know it's here in our area, and we aren't looking for it like we need to be. It's maddening."[17]

There are two types of COVID tests: Tests for the acute infection and tests for antibodies one develops after the infection.

Testing for the acute infection. This generally involves taking a sample from the nasopharynx. Saliva also has been used for this test. The test looks for genetic material, typically viral RNA, using a technique called reverse transcription polymerase chain reaction (RT-PCR). Viral RNA is detected within the first day or two of symptoms and typically peaks within the first week.[18] Viral detection then fades and usually is undetectable by three weeks.

The PCR test is used to determine active infection, our best way to detect persistent shedding of the virus and potential transmissibility. The accuracy of this test varies based on the assay used, the adequacy of the specimen, the site the specimen was obtained from and the duration of the infection at the time of testing. At the first sign of infection the test is positive in only 30-50 percent of people but that positive rate is much higher after 2-4 days of symptoms. That is the best time to perform a test for the acute infection but still it may have a 20-30 percent false negative rate.

Since PCR testing for acute infection depends on timing of the test and can have up to 30 percent false negatives, any individual should be considered to be infected if their symptoms are consistent with acute COVID infection.

---

[17] Primary Care Collaborative. Quick COVID-19 Primary Care Survey. April 24, 2020.

[18] Sethuraman N, et al Interpreting diagnostic tests for SARS-CoV-2. *JAMA*. May 6, 2020.

The initial CDC guidelines suggested that people with confirmed or presumed infection should remain in isolation for at least seven days from symptom onset and return to work once they are asymptomatic for 72 hours.

What about people who continue to test positively for the acute infection? A report from Mt. Sinai Hospital in New York found that 20 percent of people had persistently positive nasopharyngeal tests for two weeks or longer after their symptoms had completely resolved.[19] We aren't certain if this positivity indicates that the virus is still truly infectious since the test may be picking up inert viral genetic fragments. It is known that in measles and Ebola the virus can show up in tests for months related to these genetic fragments without evidence of infectivity.

Andrew Joseph, writing for *STAT* on April 20 noted, "The tests used to diagnose Covid-19 look for snippets of the virus' genome, its RNA. But what they can't tell you is if what they're finding is evidence of "live" virus, meaning infectious virus. Once a person fights off a virus, viral particles tend to linger for some time. These cannot cause infections, but they can trigger a positive test. The levels of these particles can fluctuate, which explains how a test could come back positive after a negative test. But it does not mean the virus has become active, or infectious, again. And two: the diagnostic tests typically rely on patient samples pulled from way back in their nasal passages. Collecting that specimen is not foolproof. Testing a sample that was improperly collected

---

[19] Wajnberg A, et al. Humoral immune response and prolonged PCR positivity in a cohort of 1343 SARS-CoV 2 patients in the New York City region. medRxiv. *BMJ Yale* 2020. https://doi.org/10.1101/2020.

could lead to a negative test even if the person has the virus. If that patient then gets another test, it might accurately show they have the virus."[20]

Testing blood for antibodies that we form in response to the infection. These antibodies take days to weeks to develop and therefore are not used in detecting acute infection. IgM antibodies are usually detectable during the first week and IgG antibodies at 7 to 21 days after the initial symptoms.

Testing for the antibody to COVID-19 can potentially determine individual and population immunity. It is also the best way to test people late in the acute illness, such as after two weeks of symptoms. At that late date the PCR test will likely turn negative. However,

a. We don't yet know if the antibody test is a reliable marker of immunity.

b. We don't know what level of antibody correlates with immunity.

c. We can't tell how long immunity lasts.

This later question is especially vexing since immunity for infections can last a lifetime, as is the case for measles, or it can be very fleeting. Mark Lipsitch, an epidemiologist at Harvard, modeled COVID immunity to that known from earlier studies of related coronavirus outbreaks (SARS and MERS) and concluded that, "After being infected with SARS-CoV-2, most individuals will have an immune response, some better than others. That

---

[20] Andrew Joseph. Everything we know about coronavirus immunity and antibodies-and plenty we still don't. *STAT*. April 20, 2020.

response, it may be assumed, will offer some protection over the medium term—at least a year—and then its effectiveness might decline. If it is true that infection creates immunity in most or all individuals and that the protection lasts a year or more, then the infection of increasing numbers of people in any given population will lead to the buildup of so-called herd immunity. If herd immunity is widespread enough, then even in the absence of measures designed to slow transmission, the virus will be contained — at least until immunity wanes or enough new people susceptible to infection are born."[21]

A study from Mt. Sinai Hospital in New York evaluated almost 600 people thought clinically to be infected. Each person was tested for both the acute infection, with nasopharyngeal PCR, and for subsequent immunity, with serum IgG antibodies.[22] Only 3 percent of those 600 individuals had been seen in the ER or hospitalized, so most had mild COVID infection. More than 99 percent of the patients with acute COVID infection, determined either by PCR positive tests or by a clinical picture consistent with acute COVID, had developed IgG antibodies. These antibodies were present over a period of 7 to 50 days from symptom onset and 5 to 49 days from symptom resolution. Based on this time frame, the investigators suggested that antibody testing should wait until at least three to four weeks after symptoms begin. Patient age, gender or symptom duration did not correlate with antibody response. Dr. Florian Krammer, a virologist at Mount Sinai, noted, "So everyone who makes

---

[21] Mark Lipsitch. Who is immune to the Coronavirus? *New York Times*. April 13, 2020.
[22] Wajnberg

27

antibodies is likely to have some immunity to the virus. I'm fairly confident about this."[23]

The antibody test also can have false positives and negatives. False positive tests would be particularly hazardous when deciding who is safe to return to work, as many countries are banking on. Dr. Krammer cautioned, "You don't want anybody back to work who has a false positive — that's the last thing you want to do." [24] Initially, many of the commercially available antibody tests were inaccurate. Until antibody testing is near 100 percent accurate, we should not grant immunity certificates, as cautioned by Persad and Emanuel, "Serology tests used to determine whether someone has had COVID-19 for licensing purposes must be valid and reliable, with high specificity and sensitivity...in the absence of a vaccine, the benefits of licenses might encourage uninfected people to relax protective measures..."[25]

We don't know how much antibody is important. Antibody tests aren't just yeah or nay but are quantitated. The more antibody that is found, the more significant that test is likely to be. Some infected patients, especially anyone who is immunocompromised, may not produce detectable antibodies. Some people, following acute COVID-19 infection, have developed very high levels of antibodies.

---

[23] Apoorva Mandavilli. After recovery from the coronavirus, most people carry antibodies. *New York Times*. May 7, 2020.
[24] *Ibid*
[25] Persad G, Emanuel EJ. The ethics of COVID-19 immunity-based licenses ("immunity passports"). *JAMA*. May 6, 2020.

Testing for acute COVID is becoming more widely available. The world-wide shortage of reliable testing for the acute infection sent everyone scurrying to develop such tests and stock up. The FDA went back and forth on their role in allowing new tests to be released to the public.[26] Then, as it became obvious that many commercial tests were faulty, the FDA reaffirmed its regulatory role. More convenient drive-through testing became the norm. The University of Florida medical school partnered with the largest senor community in the United States to set up a model for widespread PCR Covid-19 testing.[27] They were able to quickly establish large-scale, convenient field testing of more than 4000 residents of the community. A minimum of 16 testing stations were operated daily for one month and staffing included medical, pharmacy, physician assistant and nursing students. Community education and coordinated electronic scheduling and communication were important. Test results were available within three days.

The first home saliva test for acute infection was recently approved. A Q-tip style cotton nose swab is used and simply shipped to the laboratory for diagnostic testing. Testing has been developed for coronavirus antigenic particles, rather than the virus. This incorporates simpler and cheaper technology than PCR, and it may allow for much more widespread testing. Tongue, lower nasal or upper nasal swabs self-collected appear to be

---

[26] Sharfstein JM, et al. Diagnostic testing for the novel coronavirus. *JAMA*. 2020;323:1437.

[27] VandeWeerd C, et al. Patient-Centered Covid-19 Screening in a Community of Older Adults: Combining Educational and Research Components. *NEJM*. May 11, 2020.

comparable to those obtained by healthcare workers, providing greater ease and safety in obtaining samples for potential acute COVID-19 infection.[28]

There is controversy regarding the feasibility and wisdom of eventually moving to universal testing. Testing everyone in the population for acute infection is not practical if more than 95 percent of the population is negative, as is the current situation. Currently, testing for the acute infection is best reserved for at-risk populations. Antibody testing does have the potential to be used to detect so-called herd immunity and to decide when it is safe to go back to work. If nations are to make decisions based on testing, we need to test a lot more people, not just those with symptoms, and we need to make it convenient, accurate and fast. As antibody testing becomes more accurate and as more people in the population are exposed to COVID-19, antibody testing will likely be an important tool in public health decisions.[29]

Impact on Non-COVID Patients with Urgent Medical Conditions

As every health care provider and hospital have been totally focused on COVID patients, those millions of us with chronic diseases have suffered. Routine medical care was put on hold. The vast majority of health care professionals were not seeing patients in their office. We were so afraid of catching the virus, we did anything possible to avoid going to the hospital or seeing our physicians. Many people with serious health problems stayed home, fearful of

---

[28] Tu Y-P, et al. Swabs collected by patients or health care workers for SARS-CoV-2 testing. *NEJM*. June 3, 2020.

[29] Weinstein MC, et al. Waiting for certainty on Covid-19 tests-At what cost? *NEJM*. June 5, 2020.

face-to-face medical care. As a result, care for urgent medical conditions, like heart attacks and stroke, have dropped by 30-40 percent. Overall emergency department visits throughout the United States were down 50 percent in March and April.[30] In Italy during the first two months of the pandemic there was a 60 percent increase in out-of-hospital cardiac arrests compared to pre-pandemic months.[31]

Dr. Biykem Bozkurt, professor of medicine at Baylor College of Medicine said, "We are not seeing the number of patients we should be seeing. I think patients are scared to be exposed. Their perception is that hospitals are hotbeds for exposure and contamination. The complexity of cardiovascular care can become too difficult for people. Learned helplessness sets in, depression sets in, and they may give up. Please call and ask for what you need. We clinicians are here, and we want to help our patients."[32]

Dr. Reshma Gupta warned clinicians about focusing solely on COVID, "Part of the problem is seeing everything through a coronavirus lens. There are catastrophic risks when doctors and patients wear Covid-19 blinders. Stroke, heart disease, cancer, and lung diseases — among the leading causes of death in the U.S.—have not gone away just because Covid-19 has emerged. Patients and doctors are potentially missing or ignoring worrisome symptoms

[30] Wong LE, et al. Where are all the patients? *NEJM*. May 14, 2020.

[31] Baldi E, et al. Out-of-hospital cardiac arrest during the Covid-19 outbreak in Italy. *NEJM*. April 29, 2020.

[32] Usha Lee McFarling. 'Where are all our patients?: Covid phobia is keeping people with serious heart symptoms away from ERs. *STAT*. April 23, 2020.

unrelated to Covid-19 and not addressing them. Interrupting care for patients with chronic conditions can lead to disastrous outcomes."[33]

Dr. Harlan Krumholz, a cardiologist at Yale New Haven Hospital asked, "Where are all the patients with heart attacks and stroke? They are missing from our hospitals…cardiologists are seeing a 40 percent to 60 percent reduction in admissions for heart attacks…We actually expected to see more heart attacks during this time. Respiratory infections typically increase the risk of heart attacks. Also, times of stress increase the risk of heart attacks and strokes. Depression, anxiety and frustration, feelings that the pandemic might exacerbate, are all associated with a doubling or more of heart attack risks. Meanwhile, the immediate message to patients is clear: Don't delay needed treatment. If fear of the pandemic leads people to delay or avoid care, then the death rate will extend far beyond those directly infected by the virus. Time to treatment dictates the outcomes for people with heart attacks and strokes. These deaths may not be labeled Covid-19 deaths, but surely, they are collateral damage."[34]

To determine the effect of the pandemic on stroke evaluation in the United States a database of imaging studies, using MRI and ultrasounds ordered for potential strokes, was accessed. A pre-pandemic time frame of these imaging studies was compared to studies done during the early pan-

---

[33] Reshma Gupta. Collateral damage occurs when doctors and patients wear 'Covid-19 blinders'. *STAT*. May 4, 2020.

[34] Harlan M. Krumholz M.D. Where have all the heart attacks gone? *New York Times*. April 6, 2020.

demic.[35] The number of patients who underwent imaging decreased by 40 percent during the pandemic. This was seen across the country and did not vary with stroke severity, patient age or sex.

Dr. Steven Nissen, a cardiologist at the Cleveland Clinic, described a recent day in his coronary care unit when there were only seven patients, in contrast to the typical full 24-bed unit, "Where are the patients? That can't be normal. They are scared to death."[36] The inpatient stroke unit at Stanford University Medical Center, typically full with 12 to 15 patients, was empty, something that had never happened. Its director, Dr Gregory Albers said, "It's frightening. We prepared for an onslaught, but it has not arrived."[37]. Dr Richard Chazal, a past president of the American College of Cardiology, warned, "I am very, very worried that we are creating a problem that will have long-term consequences for the health of the community."[38] This problem is not confined to the United States. In a nation-wide study from Austria, during the month of March there was a 40 percent reduction in the number of hospital admissions for acute heart attacks.[39]

The COVID-19 pandemic has already had adverse consequences on life-threatening, non-infection related diseases throughout the world. In order

---

[35] Kansagra AP, et al. Collateral effect of Covid-19 on stroke evaluation in the United States. *NEJM* May 8, 2020.

[36] Gina Kolata. Amid the coronavirus crisis, heart and stroke patients go missing. *New York Times*. April 25, 2020.

[37] *Ibid*

[38] *Ibid*

[39] Metzler B. et al. Decline of acute coronary syndrome admissions in Austria since the outbreak of COVID-19: the pandemic response causes collateral damage. *Eur Heart J* April 16, 2020.

to guard against this problem continuing, the public needs to recognize that fear of COVID must not deter them from seeking care for urgent medical problems. Health care workers must reassure patients that they will be seen and cared for in a safe environment.

A community hospital in California found that in March there was a 50 percent drop in ER visits at the same time as a 45 percent increase in out of hospital cardiac arrests in their community, suggesting that patients were waiting too long to seek cardiac care.[40] They also found that their stroke patients all arrived too late to receive tissue plasminogen activator (TPA), which can dissolve blood clots and prevent the sequelae of a stroke. They then partnered with human behavior methodology experts and patients to determine the primary reasons why these patients were uniformly saying that, "the cons of getting Covid outweigh my normal health concerns." Their patient fears were summed up in three themes:

1. "Hospitals are infectious reservoirs, or as one patient noted, 'hospitals are crawling with Covid-19.'

2. Patients are not informed about the current risk-mitigation efforts at the hospital.

3. Patients need confirmation from their doctors or health system about when to go to the Emergency Department.

4. The national news focus on extreme case skews local perceptions.

---

[40] Wong, *et al*.

5. In the setting of shelter-in-place, the most vulnerable patients are disconnected."[41]

Acting on these themes, a series of messages, using social media, were designed and sent to the community to assuage unrealistic fears of coming to the hospital. The study concluded, "As we reopen the country, we may find that patients' fears of the healthcare environment extend beyond this immediate crisis. It will become increasingly important to engage the community in order to mitigate the public health risk of avoiding care for life-threatening illnesses."[42]

---

[41] *Ibid*
[42] *Ibid*

2
Risk Factors

Age and Co-morbidity

The two strongest risk factors for COVID infection and disease severity are age and existence of pre-existing medical problems, termed co-morbidities. I have both, as does just about everyone over age 65. Each morning during the past month I read the same, daily statistics about the impact that age and co-morbidities had on the outcome of patients with COVID-19 infection. In my adopted home state of Oregon, 90 percent of infection-related deaths have been in people over 65 and each person who died had a co-morbid chronic disease. Since I fit this category, how worried should I be?

The longer we are around, the more chronic diseases we get. More than 80 percent of older Americans have at least one chronic disease and 75 percent have at least two. These mainly include heart disease, stroke, diabetes and cancer, which account for two-thirds of yearly deaths.[43] Since age and multi-

---

[43] National Council on Aging. Healthy Aging Facts. 2020.

morbidity are interrelated, it is nearly impossible to tease out their individual effects.

In the United States, 80 percent of deaths from COVID have been in people over age 65. Almost all of these people are said to have, "an underlying condition." Most reports have demonstrated a COVID fatality of about 4 percent between ages 60-80 but 15 percent at age greater than 80. Looking at age effect of hospitalizations, admission to intensive care units (ICU) and deaths in multiple studies has been updated by the CDC.[44]

Age Range	Hospitalizations	Admission to ICU	Deaths
65-84	31-55%	11-33%	4-11%
85+	31-70%	6-29%	10-37%

Italy has had some of the world's highest death rates during the pandemic at 7.2 percent. Italy is the oldest country in Europe, with an average life expectancy of 82 years and 23 percent of the population is over age 65.[45] Those provinces in Italy with older average age had the greatest fatality rates. China, with a younger average age, had an overall mortality of 2.3 percent. However, every country has a similar age-related mortality trend. This is nota-

[44] CDC. Coronavirus Disease 2019. April 20, 2020.
[45] Vilpato S, et al. A Frail Health Care System for an Old Population: Lesson form the COVID-19 Outbreak in Italy. *J Gerontol.* April 21, 2020.

ble when reviewing age-related COVID-19 fatality rates from China [46] and from Italy.[47]

Age	Italy Fatality %	China Fatality %
All ages	7.2%	2.3%
40-49	0.4%	0.4%
50-59	1%	1.3%
60-69	3.5%	3.6%
70-79	13%	8%
>80	20%	15%

In every series, the vast majority of older patients who died had co-morbidities. It Italy, the mean age of the patients who died was 79 and only 1 percent of patients had no preexisting disease. The average number of co-existing diseases was three, including 36 percent with diabetes, 25 percent cardiovascular disease, and 10 percent with a history of stroke.[48] In data from China, the case fatality for patients with no underlying disease was 1 percent compared to 13 percent for those with cardiovascular disease, 9 percent with diabetes, 8 percent with hypertension and 8 percent for cancer.[49] Only 2 percent

---

[46] Wu Z, et al. Characteristics of and important lessons from the coronavirus disease 2019 (COVID-19) outbreak in China: summary of a report of 72 314 cases from the Chinese Center for Disease Control and Prevention. *JAMA.* 2020;323:1239

[47] Onder G, et al. Case-fatality rate and characteristics of patients dying in relation to COVID-19 in Italy. *JAMA.* March 23, 2020.

[48] *Ibid*

[49] Adams ML, et al. Population-Based Estimates of Chronic Conditions Affecting Risk for Complications from Coronavirus Disease, United States, *Emerg Infec Dis.* August 2020. vol 26, No 8.

of world-wide COVID-19 cases have been in children and those who have done poorly or who have died almost all had serious pre-existing chronic disease.

In a series of 2000 hospitalized COVID patients from New York, the strongest risk of hospitalization was age.[50] Patients older than 75 had a 60 times greater risk of hospitalization than patients in the 30-50 range and those 65-74 a 10 times greater risk. Co-morbidities also raised the odds of hospitalization, including 4-fold for cardiovascular disease. In 4000 COVID-19 cases seen between February 12 to March 16, 2020 80 percent of deaths were among those over 65 years.[51]

One of the largest studies involved 5700 COVID-19 patients who had been hospitalized in New York City, Long Island and Westchester County. Almost 100 percent of the patients had at least one major chronic health disorder and 88 percent had at least two.[52] Hypertension was present in 57 percent, obesity in 42 percent and diabetes in 34 percent. The case fatality rate increased with age for all patients but faster and higher for men.[53] Fewer women were hospitalized. Sixty percent of men in their 80s died compared to 48 percent of women. Case fatality for those patients who received mechanical

---

[50] Petrilli CM, et al. Factors associated with hospitalization and critical illness among 4,103 patients with COVID-19 disease in New York City. *BMJ*. April 11, 2020.

[51] MMWR. Severe outcomes among patients with coronavirus disease 2019 (COVID-19) — United States, February 12–March 16, 2020. *MMWR*. 2020;69:343.

[52] Ibid.

[53] Richardson S, et al. Presenting Characteristics, Comorbidities, and Outcomes Among 5700 Patients Hospitalized With COVID-19 in the New York City Area. *JAMA*. April 22, 2020.

ventilation was 76-97 percent in patients older than 65 years compared to 20-27 percent in those younger than 65.

The impact of age and co-morbidities on COVID is complicated. As with everything we learn about COVID-19, multiple factors intertwine in disease susceptibility, morbidity and mortality. The co-morbid risk factors so important in COVID-related severity and mortality are obesity, diabetes and hypertension, each of which are more common with age but also in certain ethnic and social economic groups. This may partly account for the increased impact of the pandemic in African American and Hispanic communities. Dr. Leora Horwitz suggests "If you're an official or city planner or hospital administrator, you want to know what to expect when the disease hits. The more disease is in the community, the more disease among people at high risk, period." [54]

The effect of aging on immunity may be a key to understanding why age is such an important risk factor for COVID complications, independent of co-morbid disease. There are many changes in immune function as we age. This includes a diminished overall immune response as well as an upregulated inflammatory response. These two immune/inflammatory age-related mechanisms are similar to what happens in COVID infected patients who develop pulmonary complications. Initially, lymphocytes (T-cells) decrease and immune

---

[54] Nadja Popovich, Anjali Singhvi, Matthew Conlen. Where chronic health conditions and coronavirus could collide. *New York Times*. May 18, 2020.

activity is slowed. This sets off compensatory inflammatory activity. In COVID inflammation this is likened to what has been called a cytokine storm, a flood of chemical mediators in an attempt to fight off the virus. Unfortunately, as often happens in immune disease, the chronic inflammation causes organ damage. It is not the virus directly damaging the lungs but rather the body's own natural resistance mechanisms going haywire. This is the reason that anti-inflammatory medications, like corticosteroids, and immuno-suppressive drugs, used to treat rheumatoid arthritis, have been tried in hospitalized and seriously ill COVID patients.

Age-related influences in immunity are also important in vaccine development. [55] Generally, vaccine protection decreases with age, but this varies tremendously among certain people and with specific vaccines. For example, the Shingrix vaccine for shingles is effective in 90 percent of people over 70. Koff and Williams concluded, "Covid-19 has highlighted the vulnerability of aging populations to emerging diseases. Far from being mere academic exercises, the answers to these questions are critical to the future of global health. The Covid-19 experience in aging populations offers a window into the profound, long-term, global demographic challenges the world is facing. According to the United Nations, projections indicate that by 2050 there will be more than twice as many people over 65 as there are children under 5, and the number of people 65 years of age or older globally will surpass the number of people 15 to 24 years of age. This global aging will create wide-spread public health challenges, dramatically increasing the burden of noncommunicable diseases and exposing our vulnerability to infectious diseases. Protecting aging populations will be a central, if not the primary, question in maintaining global health and biosecurity."[56]

Extended Care Facilities

Nursing homes have been the perfect storm setting for COVID-19 and its deadly sequelae. The same risk factors of age and co-morbidity are in play and then you add large groups of vulnerable people crowded together. It is difficult to quarantine a resident if they are sick. Caregivers move from room to room, increasing the likelihood of viral spread.

The pandemic in the United States first took hold with a single case at a skilled nursing facility in Kirkland, Washington on February 28, 2020.[57] Within three weeks, a total of 167 cases were identified, including 101 residents, 50 health care workers and 16 visitors. Thirty-four percent of the residents died. A description of a resident who died would herald that of thousands to follow: "On February 27, 2020, the facility was notified of a 73-year-old woman with cough, fever, and shortness of breath…residing where a cluster of unexplained febrile respiratory illness was occurring. The index patient had symptom onset on February 19, 2020 and worsening respiratory status requiring supplemental oxygen for 5 days before she was transferred to

---

[53] Koff WC, et al. Covid-19 and Immunity in Aging Populations — A New Research Agenda. *NEJM* April 17, 2020.

[54] *Ibid*

[57] McMichael TM, et al. Epidemiology of Covid-19 in a long-term care facility in King County, Washington. *NEJM.* 2020 Mar 27.

a local hospital on February 24. At the hospital, she was found to be febrile (temperature as high as 39.6°C), … and hypoxemic (oxygen saturation, 83 percent while she was breathing ambient air). She became more hypoxemic over the next 24 hours, despite bilevel positive airway pressure (BiPAP), and was intubated on February 25, 2020, because of respiratory failure. Her medical history included insulin-dependent type II diabetes mellitus, obesity, chronic kidney disease, hypertension, coronary artery disease, and congestive heart failure. She had no known travel or contact with persons known to have Covid-19. The patient died on March 2, 2020."[58]

By late April, there were more than 10,000 COVID-19-related nursing home deaths in the U.S. and they accounted for one-quarter of all deaths in the U.S. Gov. Andrew M. Cuomo of New York described nursing homes as a "feeding frenzy for this virus."[59] In the early phases of the pandemic, hospitals were relying on nursing homes to relieve their inpatient burden from infected patients. Patients who had recovered from COVID and were deemed stable were quickly transferred to nursing homes when home care was not available. It belatedly became clear that this was adding fuel to the fire. Cuomo noted that "nursing homes had to accept the patients— but only, he clarified, if they could do so safely. Homes unable to comply should transfer them to other facilities or notify the state Health Department."[60] Subsequently, in most parts of the

---

[58] *Ibid*

[59] Kim Barker and Amy Julia Harris. 'Playing Russian Roulette': Nursing Homes Told to Take the Infected. *New York Times*. April 24, 2020.

[60] *Ibid*

country, only certain nursing homes were designated as capable of admitting recently infected patients.

In New York, New Jersey, Massachusetts, Pennsylvania and Connecticut at least 50 percent of the COVID-related deaths have occurred in nursing homes. In some less populous states, nursing home deaths make up an even greater share of deaths, including 69 percent in Rhode Island, 64 percent in Delaware and 81 percent in West Virginia.[61] David C. Grabowski, a Harvard University researcher who studies nursing homes, predicted that eventually nursing homes will probably account for about half of all of the Covid-19 deaths in the United States. "It's in good facilities and in bad facilities. With this huge health crisis and economic downturn, we are all of a sudden seeing how risky it is to have the ownership split between the real estate side that has the most valuable asset and the operator, who is left with much less."[62] Assisted-living sites have also been hard hit although detailed statistics are not yet available.[63]

Dr. Sunil Parikh, an infectious disease specialist at Yale School of Medicine, described the all-too common scene, "It is only Saturday afternoon and our emergency department has already seen the fourth patient with Covid-19 from one of the local nursing homes this weekend. She was fine just a few days ago; now she is disoriented and can't catch her breath. At age 75 and with

---

[61] Karen Yourish, KK Rebecca Lai, Danielle Ivory, Mitch Smith. One-third of all U.S. coronavirus deaths are nursing home residents or workers. *New York Times*. May 9, 2020.

[62] Jonah Engel Bromwich, et al. New Count Reveals 1,600 More Nursing Home Deaths in N.Y. *New York Times*. May 5, 2020.

[63] Robert Weisman. Assisted-living sites struggle with coronavirus in shadow of nursing home crisis. *Boston Globe*. April 26, 2020.

other chronic conditions, should we put her on an experimental therapy? A few hours later, an ambulance brings a patient from a different nursing home, one that already has 21 residents with Covid-19 cases, three of whom died in the past week. He is 87 years old, has severe heart disease, is unresponsive, and no family member is reachable. He needs to be placed on a ventilator in order to survive, but once on the machine, his chance of getting off it alive is not great."[64] Dr. Parikh laments, "I am dismayed at the long-standing absence of a national strategic focus on nursing homes. It was not until April 30 that the Centers for Medicare and Medicaid Service announced an independent commission to focus on long-term care facilities, and the task force is not expected to meet until late May. But we've missed another important mark by not focusing on residents in long-term care facilities, as they make up the largest proportion of Covid-19 cases that are hitting our hospitals, requiring ventilation, and succumbing to the virus."[65]

It has been estimated that 44 percent of men and 58 percent of women over age 65 will use nursing homes at some time in their lives.[66] Currently 1.3 million people reside in the 15,000 US nursing homes. Long before the pandemic, the nursing home social isolation was acknowledged as a major contributor to elders' morbidity and mortality. Isolated seniors have a much greater incidence of depression and anxiety. Dr. Ken Covinsky, a geriatrician

---

[64] Du Sunil Parikh. Nursing homes, veterans' homes are national epicenters of Covid-19. *STAT*. May 8, 2020.

[65] Ibid.

[66] Barnett ML, et al. Nursing homes are ground zero for COVID-19 pandemic. *JAMA*. March 24, 2020.

at the University of California, San Francisco said, "It's not just touchy-feely stuff. Isolation is a real risk."[67] He focused on the additional, adverse pandemic effects of restricting visits from family and friends, "We have restricted something that's pretty essential. We need to move away from thinking of visitors to old people as optional."[68]

Nursing homes have long been accused of neglect and oversight. According to a 2014 report, one-third of Medicare nursing home residents suffered harm within two weeks of entry. [69] Infection control is consistently the most common violation cited at nursing homes. There are 1-3 million serious nursing home infections yearly. The COVID pandemic has greatly intensified the need to improve the substandard care at many nursing homes.

Federal nursing home standards need to be enforced. These should include infection control measures[70] as well as general staffing upgrades:[71]

- Standardized procedures to assure adequate hygiene, sanitization
- Necessary protective equipment
- Adequate testing capabilities
- Strict patient and staff screening
- Separate facility for infected residents
- Minimum of 4.1 hours of daily care per resident

---

[67] Paula Span. Just what older people didn't need: more isolation. *New York Times*. April 13, 2020.
[68] Ibid.
[69] Richard Mollot. Nursing homes were a disaster waiting to happen. *New York Times*. April 28, 2020.
[70] Parikh
[71] Mollot

- Minimum of one RN each shift

A group of critical care doctors who have treated COVID-19 patients have urged nursing homes to do pulse oximetry checks daily, and twice daily in any facility with known infections.[72] They commented, "We are emergency and I.C.U. doctors who have worked in three hothouses of the Covid-19 pandemic: Northern Italy, New York City and Miami. Treating scores of critically ill patients, we all observed similar patterns: Many of the patients we saw in our emergency rooms had advanced cases of Covid-19 pneumonia when they arrived — and many of those critically ill patients came from nursing homes. How then do we identify patients with Covid-19 pneumonia earlier so that they can be treated before requiring a ventilator? Clinicians have a universally available, quick and remarkably effective tool to detect the attack on the lungs caused by Covid-19 pneumonia: pulse oximetry."[73]

Residents in extended care facilities have been particularly affected by isolation and quarantine, not able to see their families and loved ones. Goldie Albertson, a 79-year old nursing home resident complained, "It does kind of get boring once in a while. I remember when the polio came out, it wasn't like this. We weren't locked up in our homes. We can't leave the building right now

---

[72] Richard Levitan, Nicholas Caputo, Roberto Cosentini, Jorge Cabrera. We Treated Older Coronavirus Patients. Here's How to Save More of Them. *New York Times.* May 10, 2020.

[73] Ibid.

with this crazy virus. It's the same way, all the time. It is hard. It's hard when you can't go anywhere."[74]

Dr. Louise Aronson noted, "I'm acutely aware of the perverse poignancy with which the outsized impact of Covid-19 on elders has laid bare medicine's outdated, frequently ineffective or injurious approach to the care of patients who are the planet's fastest-growing age group and the generations most often requiring health care. The Centers for Disease Control and Prevention did not create a Covid-19 Web page directed to elders until mid-March, nearly 2 months after we learned of that group's extraordinarily high risk for critical illness and death. Most medical centers have protocols for children and adults, but nothing for elders. Basic standards of health equity demand protocols with elder-specific diagnostic, treatment, and outcome-prediction tools, addressing lower baseline and illness-related body temperatures, atypical disease presentations, and care options geared to the life stage, health status, and life expectancy of older patients."[75]

Healthcare Workers

Healthcare workers have been on the frontline since day one of the pandemic. Dr. Li Weinlang, one of the first physicians to alert the public to the lurking COVID-pandemic, died from the infection on February 6. His sudden death spurred an online revolt in China over government attempts to silence his early warnings.

---

[74] Elliot Ross, Amelia Nierenberg. It's hard when you can't go anywhere: Life inside an assisted living facility. *New York Times*. May 9, 2020.

[75] Louse Aronson, MD. Age, Complexity, and Crisis — A Prescription for Progress in Pandemic. *NEJM* April 7, 2020.

Although there have been no official reports of fatality rates in health-care workers, on, May 8, 2020 an international list of more than 1000 doctors who died from COVID-19 was released.[76] On March 30, Italy reported that 61 doctors and healthcare workers had died from COVID-19.[77] Most were from northern Italy, the epicenter in Italy and 38 percent were primary care providers. Dr. Filippo Anelli, president of the country's National Federation of Orders of Surgeons and Dentists said, "Our doctors have been sent to war unarmed. The dead do not make a noise. Yet, the names of our dead friends, our colleagues, put here in black and white, make a deafening noise."[78]

By mid-March 3300 healthcare workers in China had been infected and 20 percent of healthcare workers in Italy had been infected.[79] Healthcare workers everywhere have been quarantined after being exposed or getting the virus. In the same section of Northern Italy with the 61 deaths in March there were many doctors testing positive and 80 healthcare workers under quarantine.[80] Dr. Stephen Anderson, a physician for 35 years in Seattle, sent his wife to their mountain cabin, noting, "I am sort of a pariah in my family. I haven't slept for longer than three hours in the past two weeks. Most physicians

---

[76] In Memoriam: Healthcare Workers Who Have Died of COVID-19. *Medscape.* May 8, 2020.

[77] Zosia Chustecka. More than 60 doctors in Italy have dies in COVID-19 pandemic. *Medscape.* March 30, 2020.

[78] Ibid.

[79] Editorial. COVID-19: protecting health-care workers. *The Lancet.* 2020;395:922.

[80] Karen Weise. Doctors Fear Bringing Coronavirus Home: 'I Am Sort of a Pariah in My Family'. *New York Times.* March 16, 2020.

have never seen this level of angst and anxiety in their careers. I am dipping myself into the swamp every day."[81]

After two emergency medicine physicians were noted to be in critical condition, Dr. William Jaquis, the head of the American College of Emergency Physicians warned, "A lot of us think that despite everything we do, we will probably be exposed. The first reported case certainly sends a shock wave through the community."[82]

One of the thousands of healthcare workers who travelled to New York to help out at the peak of the pandemic, Paul Cary, a 66-year old retired paramedic and firefighter from Colorado, died from COVID on May 1. He had already signed up for a second 30-day deployment in New York when he began to feel ill. New York Mayor, Bill de Blasio, paid tribute to Cary, "We have lost someone who came to our aid, to our defense, and there's something particularly painful when someone does the right thing—a fellow American comes from across the country to try to help the people of New York City, and while working to save lives here, gives his own life. It's very painful."[83]

In the coming months it is likely that the morbidity and mortality faced by healthcare workers from COVID-19 infection will continue to grow. Healthcare workers will also be at great risk for enduring mental health

---

[81] Ibid.

[82] Karen Weise. Two emergency room doctors are in critical condition with coronavirus. *New York Times*. March 15, 2020.

[83] Jenny Gross. Colorado paramedic who came to help New York dies from Covid-19. *New York Times*. May 2, 2020.

challenges from the overwhelming stress of the pandemic, to be discussed in a subsequent chapter.

Obesity and diabetes

Other than age and co-mortality, obesity and diabetes are the most important risk factors for poor outcome from COVID infection. Like age and multi-morbidity, it is virtually impossible to disentangle obesity from Type 2 diabetes. Nevertheless, they both have an impact on COVID morbidity and mortality.

Obesity was present in 42 percent of 5700 Covid-19 patients from New York City, Long Island and Westchester.[84] Another report from New York City of more than 4000 patients treated at NYU Langone Medical Center from March 1 to April 2, 2020 found that if patients had a body mass index (BMI) greater than 40, they had a 6-fold greater risk of hospitalization than normal weight COVID-patients.[85] BMI is defined as the body mass or weight, in kilograms (kg), divided by the square of the body height, in meters, and expressed in kg/m². Obese is generally considered to be a BMI of 30-35, moderately to severely obese 35-40 and > 40, very severely obese. Obesity was a significantly higher risk factor than for cardiovascular or pulmonary disease. Dr. Leora Horwitz, the senior author of that paper noted, "Obesity is more

---

[84] Richardson S, et al. Presenting Characteristics, Comorbidities, and Outcomes Among 5700 Patients Hospitalized With COVID-19 in the New York City Area. *JAMA*. 2020. Apr 22.

[85] Petrilli CM, et al. Factors associated with hospitalization and critical illness among 4,103 patients with Covid-19 disease in New York City. *medRxiv* preprint. https://doi.org/10.1101/2020.04.08.20057794

important for hospitalization than whether you have high blood pressure or diabetes, though these often go together, and it's more important than coronary disease or cancer or kidney disease, or even pulmonary disease. It means that as clinicians, we should be thinking a little more carefully about those patients with obesity when they come in—we should worry about them a little bit more." [86] Dr Roy Gulick, Chief of Infectious Diseases at Weill Cornell Medical Center, agreed and commented, "If obesity does turn out to be an important risk factor for younger people, and we look at the rest of the United States—where obesity rates are higher than in New York—that will be of great concern. We may see a lot more younger people being hospitalized."[87]

In 124 COVID-19 patients admitted to an ICU in France obesity was present in 48 percent and severe obesity in 28 percent.[88] The need for mechanical ventilation correlated with these patients' BMI and this was independent of diabetes. Obese patients had a seven times greater risk for needing mechanical ventilation than normal weight patients. Another report from a different French province found a lower prevalence, 11 percent, of obesity in their ICU COVID patients.[89] The authors attributed this difference

---

[86] Roni Caryn Rabin. Obesity Linked to Severe Coronavirus Disease, Especially for Younger Patients. *New York Times.* April 16, 2020.

[87] Ibid.

[88] Simonnet A, et al. High prevalence of obesity in severe respiratory syndrome coronavirus-2 (SARS-CoV19) requiring invasive mechanical ventilation. *Obesity.* April 9, 2020.

[89] Caussy C, et al. Obesity is associated with severe forms of COVID-19. *Obesity.* April 21, 2020.

to a lower background rate of obesity in that province. They also found a high requirement for mechanical ventilation in the COVID patients with severe obesity.

Diabetes has been a strong risk factor for COVID infection and severity of infection in reports from every country. Most reports do not distinguish between type 1 and type 2 diabetes although about 90 percent of cases world-wide are type 2. In a systematic analysis of nine studies from China, three was a three-fold risk of infection and infection severity for patients with diabetes.[90] The case fatality rate in China for 72,000 people infected with COVID was 2 percent but 7.3 percent for patients with diabetes.[91] The only co-morbidity with a higher fatality rate in their patients was cardiovascular disease. Diabetes was present in 36 percent of COVID patients hospitalized in Italy and 34% who died.[92] Diabetes has also been a risk factor for prior coronavirus-related epidemics, including the Middle East Respiratory Syndrome (MERS-CoV) in 2012.[93]

---

[90] Chen Y, et al. Effects of hypertension, diabetes and coronary heart disease on COVID-19 diseases severity: a systematic review and meta-analysis. https://www.medrxiv.org/content/10.1101/2020.03.25.2004313.

[91] Wu C, et al. Risk factors associated with acute respiratory distress syndrome and death in patients with coronavirus disease 2019 pneumonia in Wuhan, China. *JAMA Intern Med*. March 13, 2020.

[92] Onder G, et al. Case-fatality rate and characteristics of patients dying in relation to COVID-19 in Italy. *JAMA*. 2020. Mar 23.

[93] Badawi A, et al. Prevalence of comorbidities in the Middle East respiratory syndrome coronavirus (MERS-CoV): a systematic review and meta-analysis. *Int J Infect Dis* 2016:49;129.

Obesity and diabetes alter immunity. This can be detected initially in adipose tissue with excess cytokine release.[94] Left unchecked, this leads to insulin resistance, even before diabetes is diagnosed. Even short-term increases in blood sugar alter immunity and inhibit normal microbial killing.[95] Studies have demonstrated that optimal blood sugar control reduces infection rate and its complications. eventually promoting inflammation and insulin resistance.[96] Diabetes may also enhance viral entry into cells and a study of 161 COVID patients from Wuhan, China found that those with diabetes had delayed viral clearing.[97]

The COVID-19 pandemic has been on a collision course with America's growing epidemic of obesity and diabetes, both serious diseases in their own right. Dr. Matthew Hutter, president of the American Society for Metabolic and Bariatric Surgery reminds us that "We in the U.S. have not always identified obesity as a disease, and some people think it's a lifestyle choice. But it's not. It makes people sick, and we're realizing that now."[98]

The U.S. has the highest obesity rate among countries with an advanced health-care system. The prevalence of obesity is significantly greater in the U.S. than China and Italy, other countries hit hard by the pandemic. Our obesity rate is four-fold higher that Norway and Switzerland. Obesity in the U.S. has

---

[94] Shu CJ, et al. The immune system's involvement in obesity-driven type 2. *Diabetes Semin Immunol* 2012;24:436.

[95] Jafar N, et al. The effect of short-term hyperglycemia on the innate immune system. *Am J Med Sci* 2016;351:201.

[96] Ibid.

[97] Chen X, et al. Hypertension and diabetes delay the viral clearance in COVID-19 patients. medRxiv. 2020 .20040774

[98] Rabin, 2020.

increased by 600 percent since the 1980s.[99] Currently 42 percent of the US population are classified as obese and 8 percent as severely obese.[100] It is estimated that by 2030 almost one-half of Americans will be obese and one-fourth severely obese. The BMI correlates with mortality rate, particularly that related to cardiovascular disease. The average survival for people with a BMI between 30-35 is reduced by 2-4 years and by 8-10 years for a BMI at 40-45.[101] Eleven percent of Americans, 35 million of us, have diabetes. In those over age 60, that percentage goes up to 27 percent.[102] Over the past 20 years there has been a parallel increase in childhood obesity and type 2 diabetes. Obesity, diabetes and hypertension together greatly increase cardiovascular complications and decrease overall survival.

Physicians and the public must recognize that obesity and diabetes increase the risk of COVID-19 infection and disease severity. In any patient with COVID infection, optimal blood glucose control is most important. Hyperglycemia may adversely affect pulmonary function and immune response. Blood glucose should be carefully monitored. Since diabetes and hypertension often coexist, it is important that blood pressure be well-

---

[99] Flegal KM, et al. Trends in obesity among adults in the United States, 2005 to 2014. *JAMA*. 2016;315:22841

[100] Scott Hahan. Practical strategies for engaging individuals with obesity in primary care. *Mayo Clin Proc*. 2018;93:351.

[101] Price GM, et al. Weight, shape, and mortality risk in older persons: elevated waist-hip ratio, not high body mass index, is associated with a greater risk of death. *Am J Clin Nutr*. 2006; 84:449.

[102] American Diabetes Association. Comprehensive Medical Evaluation and Assessment of Comorbidities: Standards of Medical Care in Diabetes-2020. *Diabetes Care*. 2020;43(Suppl 1):S37.

controlled. Initially there was concern that certain blood pressure medications, especially angiotensin-converting enzyme (ACE) inhibitors, might lead to worse infection but that has not been confirmed. There should be a low threshold for hospitalization when patients with diabetes and obesity become infected with COVID-19.

Immunosuppression

When the pandemic first struck, any patient considered to be immune compromised was considered to be at high risk of getting infected and for complications from COVID infection. It turns out to be more complicated than that generalization.

Some immune diseases or the medications used to treat them do lower resistance to infections below the breaking point. This is the situation for certain forms of cancer. Early studies did reveal a significant increased fatality rate among COVID-19 patients with cancer.[103] In these situations, the risk of COVID-19 infection needs to be balanced against the risk of delaying or changing cancer therapy. Some cancers, such as acute leukemia or advanced lymphoma, are quickly lethal and chemotherapy can't be delayed.

Dr. Urvi Shah, an oncologist who also has Hodgkin's lymphoma, described his dilemma when he got COVID-19 infection, "Given my cancer history, I could not help but wonder if my immune system had returned to its baseline and if I would be able to weather this infection without serious comp-

---

[103] Liang W, et al. Cancer patients in SARS-CoV-2 infection: a nationwide analysis in China. *Lancet Oncol.* 2020;21:335.

lications. Would I need to be admitted to the hospital? Would I need to go to the intensive care unit? Would the prior chemotherapy affect my current outcomes? As an oncologist and a cancer survivor, I also worried about the patients for whom I was caring. Asking the average person to stay at home and put their life on pause for a few weeks to months can sound like a reasonable measure to take to curb this pandemic. But that is not an option for many patients with cancer receiving active lifesaving therapy. So these patients must go to war every day with both cancer and COVID-19—and every patient's trip to the chemotherapy suite to extend their life has the potential to abruptly shorten it."[104]

What about immune/rheumatic diseases? Being a rheumatologist, I have been very concerned with the potential for an increased risk of COVID infection for my patients. We know that immune/rheumatic diseases and the medications we use to treat them can increase the risk of infection. Our patients hear such warnings constantly, since each consumer pitch on television for the latest drug to treat rheumatoid arthritis, psoriasis or inflammatory bowel disease cautions about tuberculosis, bacterial or fungal infections.

Studies by many of my rheumatology colleagues have shed light on just how worried we should be. The early answer is that patients with immune diseases who are stable should continue on their current management. It is most important to keep their immune disease under good control. If the underlying disease flares up, subsequent tissue and systemic inflammation will serve as a

---

[104] Shah UA. Cancer and coronavirus disease 2019 (COVID-19)-facing the "C words". *JAMA Oncol.* May 7, 2020.

potent nidus for infection. In patients exposed to the virus but not infected, immunosuppressive medications should be stopped temporarily, pending a negative test for infection or a two-week symptom free period. However, if a patient has a confirmed or suspected infection, immunosuppressive medications should be held until the patient has fully recovered.

Rheumatologists from the United Kingdom, Australia and a number of other countries have come to the same conclusions. There is no evidence that the risk of COVID infection or its sequelae are directly related to a specific disease, such as rheumatoid arthritis or systemic lupus erythematosus. Rather, the risk is related to the general factors we have discussed, namely age and co-morbidity. In 86 patients with various immune/inflammatory diseases from New York there was no greater risk of hospitalization compared to infected patients from the general population.[105] In a report from Lombardy, Italy, only 8 of 320 rheumatic disease patients, like rheumatoid arthritis, had been diagnosed with COVID-19 infection, despite that area being hard hit by the pandemic.[106]

The infection risk of immunosuppressive medications varies with each drug's mechanism of action as well as the dose used. On one end of the spectrum are medications used for cancer chemotherapy, some of which can lower white blood cell counts precipitously. In contrast, many of the drugs used

---

[105] Haberman R, et al. Immune-mediated inflammatory diseases-Case series from New York. *NEJM*. Apr 29, 2020.
[106] Monti S, et al. Clinical course of COVID-19 in a series of patients with chronic arthritis treated with immunosuppressive targeted therapies. *Ann Rheum Dis* 2020; 79:667.

to treat rheumatic and other immune diseases, such as non-steroidal anti-inflammatory drugs, like ibuprofen or naproxen, have no significant immune effect. The antimalarials, including hydroxychloroquine (*plaquenil*), methotrexate and sulfasalazine, have minimal immune effects. None of these drugs need to be stopped or changed, even if a patient becomes infected.

There is some evidence, and a lot of media attention, for the potential beneficial therapeutic role in COVID infection of certain antirheumatic and immunosuppressive medications. This became an international issue after President Donald Trump announced that antimalarials may be effective against COVID infection, and "since they are cheap and available, why not try them?".[107] Dr. Anthony Fauci, Director of the National Institute of Allergy and Infectious Disease, and other medical experts noted that any benefit from these medications was anecdotal and subsequent controlled studies have demonstrated no obvious efficacy from antimalarial medications, with adverse side effects.[108]

There are potential benefits from using powerful immunosuppressive medications when COVID patients become seriously ill. Many of the COVID complications, including the lung injury, are related to immune and anti-inflammatory mechanisms, often called the "cytokine storm". High doses of corticosteroids and certain immunosuppressive medications have been tried throughout the world in critically ill COVID patients. Until more evidence

[107] Thomas K, Grady D. Trump's embrace of unproven drugs to treat coronavirus defies science. *The New York Times*. March 20, 2020.
[108] Geleris J, et al. Observational study of hydroxychloroquine in hospitalized patients with Civid-19. *NEJM*. May 7, 2020.

comes to light, it is recommended that these medications only be used in controlled, clinical trials.

There are similar recommendations for the treatment of other immune diseases during the COVID pandemic. Guidelines for the treatment of ulcerative colitis and Crohn's disease[109], psoriasis[110] and multiple sclerosis[111] reflect those for rheumatic diseases and follow the same basic principles:

- If stable, continue on current medications.
- Avoid disease flare-ups, whenever possible.
- Frequent monitoring for infection.
- If contact with suspected or confirmed infection, self-isolate and hold any immunosuppressive medication.
- If infected, hold all immunosuppressive medications. Low index of suspicion for hospitalization.

In the near future we will be able to better advise patients with immune diseases on their risk from COVID infection. There will be available data to better inform physicians and their patients whether certain immunosuppressants may be riskier and, hopefully, whether certain of these medications may be effective in treating its complications.

---

[109] Mao R, et al. Implications of COVID-19 for patients with pre-existing digestive diseases. *Lancet Gastroenterol Hepatol.* 2020 Mar 11

[110] Price KN, et al. COVID-19 and immunomodulator/immunosuppressant use in dermatology. *J Am Acad Dermatol* 2020. May:82:e173.

[111] Willis MD, et al. Multiple sclerosis and the risk of infection. *J Neurol.* 2020;267:1567.

3
Initial Healthcare Response

Primary care

The COVID-19 pandemic quickly and dramatically changed every aspect of primary care medicine. Most primary care offices throughout the country were near-empty for the first few months after the pandemic took hold. Primary care health providers, as well as specialists, followed the public health guidelines for social distancing, limiting patient contact largely to telephone calls and, when available, virtual health-care visits. Patients were told to avoid any non-emergent appointments. Instead of seeing their primary care providers (PCP), people were forced to seek medical advice over the phone. During the months of March and April, more than 80 percent of primary care visits were solely by telephone. Patients who typically saw their PCP regularly were told to hold-off a few weeks or months for their next blood pressure or blood sugar test and to self-monitor.

This initial response to the COVID-19 pandemic put primary care in the United States under extraordinary financial pressure. On April 2, 2020 a survey of 3000 PCPs reported that 90 percent of PCPs had stopped routine patient check-ups.[112] Two-thirds of the PCPs said that they were uncertain whether their practice would be open in a few months and 80 percent described their practice as under severe fiscal strain as a result of the COVID-19 pandemic. An April 27 update of that survey found that 70 percent were not having face-to-face patient visits and 50 percent of PCPs had laid off or furloughed staff.[113] Those PCPs that were billing for virtual healthcare visits were receiving less than one-half of their normal face-to-face visits.

Dr. Daniel Horn, a PCP and director of population health at Massachusetts General Hospital, spoke to one primary care doctor at a small practice who said: "This is profoundly depressing. I have worked my whole life to serve my community, and I don't see how I can keep my practice running for another eight weeks." [114] Horn and colleagues suggested "immediate financial relief to primary care practices by switching from fee for service to a monthly bundled payment…provide all primary care practices nationwide with a reasonable fixed payment, say on average $50 per patient per month, retroactive to April 1 and through the end of 2020. This fixed payment would replace any previous fee-for-service payments the practice would have received during this time. Practices that serve patients with greater health needs

[112] Primary Care Collaborative. Quick Ovid-19 Primary Care Survey. April 2, 2020
[113] Primary Care Collaborative. Quick Ovid-19 Primary Care Survey. April 27, 2020
[114] Daniel Horn, Wayne Altman, Zirui Song. Primary care is being devastated by Covid-19. It must be saved. *STAT.* April 29, 2020.

could receive a larger budget than those that serve healthier patients, a risk-adjustment process used by most public and private payers today."[115]

Horn also noted that nationally healthcare saw a 55-70 percent decrease in revenue since the start of the pandemic and worried that, "…a reckoning is coming. Half of all family medicine physicians work in small practices that aren't cross subsidized by other lucrative specialties. Instead, they rely on high volumes and minor procedures. At Northampton Area Pediatrics, a 40-year-old primary-care clinic in western Massachusetts, volume has plummeted during the pandemic. 'What was a day typically spent seeing upwards of 30-plus kids became seeing anywhere from 8 to 15 children on telemedicine,' says pediatrician Ryan Kearney, who works there. His bosses applied for, but did not receive, a Payroll Protection Program loan. They've had to lay off a third of the workforce, including front-desk staff, medical assistants, nurses, a physician and two nurse practitioners. David Steele, the managing partner, worries, 'We will never return to the world we had.'"[116]

Dr. Farzad Mostashari, a former health officer in the Barack Obama administration, commented, "Our doctors are telling their patients, don't come into the office, which means that the offices are not making any money. They're really, really worried about how many weeks they can last before they literally have to shut their doors at a time when we need that frontline capacity. We have to pay special attention to these independent primary care

---

[115] *Ibid*
[116] Daniel Horn. The pandemic could put your doctor out of business. *The Washington Post*. April 24, 2020.

practices."[117] Michael Chernow, a health policy professor at Harvard Medical School said, "I worry about how well these practices will be able to shoulder the financial burden to be able to meet the health care needs people have. If practices close down, you lose access to a point of care."[118]

As practices are gradually opening up, scheduling changes become more complicated. Many practices are already scheduling well-patient visits only on specific half-days. One of the most challenging aspects will be to catch-up with routine care and, most importantly, immunizations.

Dr. Sean O'Leary, a member of the American Academy of Pediatrics Committee on Infectious Diseases told *The New York Times* on April 23, 2020: "The last thing we want as the collateral damage of Covid-19 are outbreaks of vaccine-preventable diseases, which we will almost certainly see if there continues to be a drop in vaccine uptake."[119] A pediatric electronic health records company reported that for the week of April 5, the administration of measles, mumps and rubella immunizations fell by 50 percent compared to pre-pandemic weeks.[120] Diphtheria and whooping cough shots decreased by 42 percent and HPV vaccines by 73 percent.

---

[117] Reed Abelson. Doctors without patients: Our waiting rooms are like ghost towns. *New York Times*. May 5, 2020.
[118] Ibid.
[119] Jan Hoffman. Vaccine Rates Drop Dangerously as Parents Avoid Doctor's Visits. *New York Times*. April 23, 2020.
[120] *Ibid*

Telemedicine

The COVID-19 pandemic has thrust telemedicine into the frontline of every hospital and medical practice. Almost overnight, the pandemic forced doctors to close their offices and shift almost exclusively to telemedicine. In 2019, only 8 percent of American healthcare was using telemedicine.[121] Both patients and health care providers were uncomfortable with the technology and saw no compelling reason to replace in-person care with virtual care. During the months of March and April 2020, more than 80 percent of US primary care visits were by telephone.[122]

Telemedicine, also referred to as telehealth, uses technology to provide healthcare at a distance. Telemedicine includes telephone visits, video visits and remote patient monitoring. The main use of telehealth during the first wave of the pandemic was via telephone visits. Telephone visits are the simplest form of telemedicine, universally available at low cost to providers. As the pandemic began, telemedicine was the only practical and safe way to answer the unending questions about potential infection, testing and to begin triaging. Patients experienced very long telephone-hold times and delayed message responses.

Dr. Stephen Parodi, an infectious disease specialist predicted, "The use of telemedicine is going to be critical for management of this pandemic. Many of them don't want to come in and be exposed in a clinic or office setting. The

---

[121] AmericanWell. Amwell Telehealth Index: 2019 Consumer Survey 2019. March 30, 2020.
[122] Primary Care Collaborative.

patients have been appreciative of that switch."[123] Dr. Peter Antall, the chief medical officer for a company working with health systems across the country said, "Telehealth is being rediscovered. Everybody recognizes this is an all hands-on deck moment. We need to scale up wherever we can."[124]

Dr. Sam Wessely, a general practitioner in London said "We're basically witnessing 10 years of change in one week. It used to be that 95 percent of patient contact was face-to-face: You go to see your doctor, as it has been for decades, centuries. But that has changed completely."[125]

Drs. Ezekiel Emanuel and Amol Navathe, who direct the Healthcare Transformation Institute at the University of Pennsylvania noted, "Telemedicine is now everywhere. For years doctors resisted telemedicine, either because it was too hard to learn or, worse, because they made more money from an in-office visit. Last year just 22 percent of family physicians surveyed used video visits, according to the American Academy of Family Physicians. This is crucial because telemedicine is cost-efficient for matters that do not need physical contact and easier to work into patients' daily life, and it frees up office visits for patients with complex conditions. It also makes it easier for doctors to provide after-hours care, reducing costly emergency room and urgent care clinic visits."[126]

---

[123] Reed Abelson. Doctors and patients turn to telemedicine in the coronavirus outbreak. *New York Times*. March 11, 2020.

[124] *Ibid*

[125] Benjamin Mueller. Telemedicine arrives in the U.K.: '10 years of change in one week'. *New York Times*. April 5, 2020.

[126] Ezekiel J Emanuel, Amol S Navathe. Will 2020 be the year that medicine was saved? *New York Times*. April 14, 2020.

The pandemic pushed telemedicine into the frontline of health care throughout the world. Within a matter of weeks, hospitals and physician practices were exclusively using telemedicine to field all COVID-related questions, to coordinate testing and to triage clinical care.[127] Medical offices used telemedicine to, "… dramatically reduce the number of nurses and physicians who physically staff the office, while other staff provide care from their home or 'clean office space… physicians are reviewing scheduled appointments and making triage decisions for in-person visits, telehealth visits, or deferred appointments."[128]

At New York University (NYU) medical center, the telehealth visits increased over 1 month from less than 1 percent of total visits to 70 percent of total visits. By May 1, all clinical staff were fully trained in inpatient and outpatient telehealth. The telehealth system was integrated with their electronic medical records, allowing scheduled outpatient video visits, virtual patient waiting rooms, scheduling and privacy/security. Pre-COVID-19, less than 50 video visits were happening in all hospital departments on a typical day. On March 19, the first day of the expanded video visits, that volume increased to more than 1,000 and reached over 7,000 visits within 10 days, or greater than 70 percent of the total ambulatory volume at this large health center.[129]

The number of telemedicine visits at the University of Pittsburgh Medical Center (UPMC) skyrocketed from 250 per day in early March to 9500

---

[127] Mehrotra A, et al. Rapidly converting to "virtual practices": Outpatient care in the era of Covid-19. *NEJM* April 1, 2020.
[128] *Ibid*
[129] *Ibid*

daily in late April, a 3700 percent increase.[130] Dr. Ravi Ramani, director of the heart failure clinic at UPMC, extolled the virtues of a video visit while seeing one of his cardiac patients, "The biggest thing I as a clinician rely on is the eyeball test. Just being able to see them, how they are sitting in their armchairs, how their skin color looks—those things are critical."

The incorporation of telemedicine is here to stay. Dr. Daniel Mann and colleagues at NYU Grossman School of Medicine predicted, "the changes instigated initially by the COVID-19 pandemic have likely irreversibly altered the position of telemedicine in the US healthcare system. When prior literature speculated about the potential primacy of telemedicine over in-person care, it seemed futuristic, but it is now a reality practiced in multiple health care systems around the world. Using telemedicine platforms, providers and patients are being forced into a new normal that includes communicating with each other through video and audio."[131]

Jane Brody, *The New York Times* medical columnist wrote, "Even if no other good for health care emerges from the coronavirus crisis, one development — the incorporation of telemedicine into routine medical care — promises to be transformative. Using technology that already exists and devices that most people have in their homes, medical practice over the internet can result in faster diagnoses and treatments, increase the efficiency of care and reduce patient stress. As the coronavirus ravaged many communities large and

---

[130] Casey Ross. In fading steel towns, chronically ill patients hope video visits stay after the pandemic goes. *STAT*. April 29, 2020.

[131] Mann DM, et al. COVID-19 transforms health care through telemedicine: evidence from the field. *Amer Med Inform Ass*. Oxford Univ Press. 2020.

small throughout the country, most patients have been unable or unwilling to access in-person care from health professionals. Even if someone is able to get to a doctor's office or clinic safely, who wants to sit in a waiting room where you or another patient might transmit the infection?"[132]

There are many glitches to work out before we commit full throttle to telemedicine. Physicians and patients worry that it is too complicated. Hollander and Sites find little evidence that telemedicine is too difficult or complicated to be universally adopted. "It turns out that when fear of catching a potentially fatal disease strikes, telemedicine is no longer too hard. Respiratory symptoms—which may be early signs of Covid-19—are among the conditions most commonly evaluated with this approach. Health care providers can easily obtain detailed travel and exposure histories. Automated screening algorithms can be built into the intake process, and local epidemiologic information can be used to standardize screening and practice patterns across providers." [133]

Since a complete physical examination cannot be performed, telemedicine cannot substitute for many aspects of an in-person examination. However, there are many aspects of an examination that can be performed virtually. Telemedicine can be depersonalizing, and clinicians are concerned that it will further dehumanize clinical care.[134] Two family doctors elegantly worried

---

[132] Jane E. Brody. A pandemic benefit: The expansion of telemedicine. *The New York Times*. May 12, 2020.

[133] Hollander JE, Carr BG. Virtually perfect? Telemedicine for Covid-19. *NEJM*. March 11, 2020.

[134] Shankar M, et al. Humanism in telemedicine: Connecting through virtual visits during the COVID-19 pandemic. *Ann Fam Med*. Posted on Covid-19 Collection. 2020.

about our loss of touch, "…at present, touch is taboo. Never entirely without risk, touch is now virally suppressed; gone. It's hands-off medicine. Face to face communication is now more than just at arm's reach…now meters away across such rooms. Virtual and video consultations are the new norm. We are in touch, but there is something missing, something evanescent…perhaps it is timely to reflect on the unspoken ways in which we relate to each other so that distance does not mean we lose touch with what define us as physician-healers. In this way, when our eyes touch, we can stay connected."[135]

Health care leaders and clinicians when asked "how will the future of health care delivery be different after this pandemic," uniformly predicted that telehealth use will be widely adopted.[136] At the time of the survey in late April, 82 percent of practices were using telemedicine for non Covid-19 medical issues, 59 percent used telemedicine to screen patients for Covid-19 and 43 percent to follow-up Covid-19 patients from ED or inpatient units. Some quotes by clinicians:[137]

- "People will be more comfortable with telehealth."
- "Telehealth has arrived."
- "We'll realize just how much care can be delivered virtually."

Quotes from clinical leaders and executives included[138]:

---

[135] Kelly MA, et al. Out of touch. *Ann Fam Med*. Posted on COVID-19 Collection. 2020.
[136] *NEJM* Catalyst. What health care leaders and clinicians say about the Covid-19 pandemic. *NEJM.* April 23, 2020.
[137] Ibid.
[138] Ibid.

- "As we determine that telemedicine is as effective as face to face encounters, and documentation requirements need not be so onerous, I expect we will adopt these changes in not pandemic times."

- "A more realistic approach to the delivery of care with broader acceptance (both from payors and providers) for innovative and virtual care delivery."

- "Needless to say, telemedicine will fill an increasing role in many management venues."

In many urban areas, PCP practices that are part of a hospital-based system have easily adapted to telemedicine. Things are much different for smaller practices, "One doctor told me they were switching from 90 percent in-person visits and 10 percent online virtual visits to the opposite, reducing their in-person visits to 10 percent of their patient encounters. Smaller practices had fewer resources to even attempt such a dramatic change. Also, salaried doctors in practices backed by large organizations were not worried about how they were going to be paid for these virtual visits or whether they could afford to keep their practice staff on payroll with dramatically declining fee-for-service income. Not so with a private practice pediatrician who was very concerned whether they were being reimbursed for telemedicine visits and worried whether they could continue to make staff payroll."[139]

---

[139] Kamerow D. Covid-19: Don't forget the impact on US family physicians. *BMJ*. 2020. doi: https://doi.org/10.1136/bmj.m1260

The majority of patients have been very appreciative of telemedicine during the early phase of the pandemic. A 36-year old pregnant woman said, "It was really nice. I felt like I had a really good connection with the doctor. I really enjoyed being able to see him and ask questions. His eyes were on the screen the majority of the time he was talking to us."[140] An 86-year old man with congestive heart failure was pleased with his telemedicine visits, "It worked out very well for the problem I was having. It's amazing. You pick up a cellphone and there's your picture and the man you're talking to. It's like he's in your living room. An awful lot of care can be done with technology. I believe this has a real future."[141]

Reimbursement for telemedicine was very poor initially. That has started to change. In March, the Centers for Medicare and Medicaid removed barriers for telemedicine compensation to equalize payments with in-person visits. Restrictions on use of remote care and administrative hurdles have eased up but remain a problem, especially for small practices. Clinicians in primary care and every specialty will need to document the impact of telemedicine on their practice in the near future.

Business as Usual?

As healthcare practices ramp back up to full operating capacity, they are being deluged with patient concerns and trying to make up for lost patient time. During the first few months of the pandemic, routine medical care was

---

[140] Casey Ross.
[141] Ibid.

put on hold. Many patients were so fearful of going to a hospital that serious medical conditions were left to fester. We have to catch up and at the same time address concerns for people with pre-existing health issues.

Dr. Barron Lerner, professor of medicine and population health at NYU Langone Medical Center lamented, "My patients continue to have medical problems that are not related to the coronavirus. But now, when I offer recommendations—especially those that possibly involve putting themselves at risk of contracting a Covid-19 infection—they often reject my advice. Given the mortality data and the constant media coverage of the Covid-19 epidemic, it is hardly surprising that my patients are freaked out about possibly becoming ill…Doctor, can't you just look up the antibiotic they gave to me last time and prescribe it? I'm afraid to go to an emergency room because I might get coronavirus." [142]

Since the pandemic began, there were no regular check-ups available for patients with high blood pressure or diabetes, the cardiovascular diseases putting us most as risk if we get COVID. In the month after the pandemic, cholesterol tests and hemoglobin A1c diabetes testing were down by 65 percent.[143] In disease epicenters like New York and Massachusetts, hemoglobin A1c and lipid panels had decreased by more than 80%.

This is exactly the time when any of us with a chronic illness need to be especially vigilant. If you already have a chronic cardiovascular disease

---

[142] Barron H Lerner MD. Weighing risks for my patients at a time of Covid-19. *New York Times*. April 30, 2020.

[143] *Komodohealth.* April 28, 2020. Routine chronic disease screenings and oncology biomarker tests plummet during COVID-19.

(CVD), be it coronary artery disease, hypertension, congestive heart failure, atrial fibrillation or another arrythmia, the physiologic stress from COVID-infection will aggravate those conditions.[144] The increased COVID-related risk is also related to the company CVD keeps, namely older age patients, often with obesity and diabetes. My cardiologist cancelled my routine atrial fibrillation check-up last month. Fortunately, I, as millions of Americans, was able to make use of digital cardiology with a remote electrocardiogram (ECG) and pacemaker check.

Treating heart disease became much more complicated during the pandemic. For example, COVID-19, like other viral diseases, may cause an acute myocarditis. This may simulate an acute heart attack with ST-segment elevation on ECG.[145] The typical blood markers for cardiac injury, including the CPK and troponin, are more difficult to evaluate since they may indicate acute heart damage but also may be elevated as part of the cytokine storm.[146]

The increase in heart attacks and stroke with COVID-19 disease suggest that excess blood clotting may be at fault. COVID patients have elevated levels of clotting factors, possibly related to the virus infecting vascular cells, causing inflammation. This is the likely explanation for an alarming number of strokes in younger people infected with COVID-19. More than 90 COVID patients with strokes were reported from China, the UK and

[144] Mehra MR, et al. Cardiovascular disease, drug therapy, and mortality in Covid-19. *NEJM.* May 1, 2020.

[145] Mahmud E, et al. Management of acute myocardial infarction during the COVID-19 pandemic. *J Am Coll Cardiol.* April 21, 2020.

[144] Li JW, et al. The impact of 2019 novel coronavirus on heart injury: A systemic review and meta-analysis. *Prog Cardiovasc Dis.* 2020. Apr 16.

France.[147] Large vessel strokes was seen during a recent 2 week stretch in five COVID-19 infected patients, each younger than age 50, at Mt Sinai Hospital in New York.[148] This led doctors there to subsequently give anticoagulant drugs to all of their hospitalized infected patients. Dr Adam Dmytriw from the University of Toronto said, "We're seeing a startling number of young people who had a minor cough, or no recollection of viral symptoms at all, and they're self-isolating at home like they're supposed to — and they have a sudden stroke."[149]

Colonoscopies, mammograms and cervical cancer screenings have been delayed since the pandemic began. As compiled by the electronic records vendor Epic, those screening appointments in March had fallen by 90% compared to previous years. The president of Epic, Carl Dvorak, worried, "We're also fairly convinced that even once they lift the lockdowns, we'll still see the concerned patients a little bit more reluctant to go in. Truthfully, it doesn't take much to talk a person out of going in for a colonoscopy."[150] He is hoping that Epic's vast network can help physicians develop a strategy for catching up and prioritizing people at high risk for missed screening. One way to address the current problem with avoiding colonoscopies is to increase the

---

[145] Elizabeth Cooney. Giving blood thinners to severely ill Covid-19 patients is gaining ground. *STAT*. May 6, 2020.

[148] Oxley TJ, et al. Large-vessel stroke as a presenting feature of Covid-19 in the young. *NEJM*. April 28, 2020.

[149] Roni Caryn Rabin. Coronavirus may pose a new risk to younger patients: Strokes. *New York Times*. May 14, 2020.

[150] Rebecca Robbins. *STAT*. May 4, 2020.

use of mailed fecal immunochemical tests. This is a simple, cheap, at-home test with good sensitivity for picking up colorectal cancer.

Cancer patients are especially vulnerable to the ravages of COVID-19 infection and have increased mortality risk.[151] This has forced oncologists to prioritize oncology care based on risk/benefit ratio, reduce hospital visits, primarily with telemedicine, and switch from intravenous infusion to oral therapy when possible.[152] [153]

In just two months, the treatment of cancer patients was transformed. As detailed by Dr. Deborah Schrag and colleagues in the April 13, *New England Journal of Medicine*, "Because some malignancies could pose an immediate threat to survival, cancer provides a lens into the major shifts currently underway in clinical care. The COVID-19 crisis is forcing elimination of low-value treatments...Many patients with cancer are concerned that their needs will be overlooked or marginalized during the COVID-19 crisis. In the space of a month, approaches and accepted norms of cancer care delivery have been transformed of necessity. Most of these changes would not have occurred without the pandemic. Although the immediate priority is to save lives, in the aftermath and recovery phase, evaluating the effects of COVID-19 on cancer mortality will be a priority. Planning for resuming cancer treatment and screening to mitigate harms is already underway. It is also likely

[151] Yang F, et al. Clinical characteristics and outcomes of cancer patients with COVID-19. *J Med Virol*. May 5, 2020.
[152] UK Coronavirus Cancer Monitoring Project Team. *Lancet Oncol.* April 15, 2020.
[153] Pramesh C.S., et al. Cancer management in India during Covid-19. *NEJM.* April 28, 2020.

that some changes provoked by the crisis will permanently transform how to treat cancer, in some cases perhaps for the benefit of both patients and their physicians."[154]

Unfortunately, adequate protective equipment was late in arriving at some oncology units. For example, Italian oncologists decried, "Our region has left us to fight the cancer battle and the COVID-19 war without true protection, without knowing whether we are infected with the virus. To stand up and fight for maintaining high standards in cancer care, we have launched a social media campaign …to extend periodical and frequent testing for SARS-CoV-2 … to health care workers involved in the treatment of patients with cancer. Our aim is to guarantee separate and "clean" pathways for patients with cancer. Even if this objective is failing in front of our very eyes, we will not give up on maintaining the involvement of institutions, patients' advocacy organizations, and oncologist associations."[155]

An oncologist at the Cleveland Clinic, Dr. Mikkael Sekeres, described his dilemma and the ordeal of one of his cancer patients since the pandemic, "But the balance of risks and benefits for all of my patient interactions has now changed. For my patients' immune systems are so exquisitely fragile, because the cancer treatments they need to fight a disease that can be scarier than Covid-19 leave them so immunosuppressed, that it doesn't take much even without a pandemic for them to catch an infection that could kill them. When I walked

---

[154] Schrag D, et al. Oncology practice during the COVID-19 pandemic. *JAMA*. April 13, 2020.

[155] Pietrantonio F, et al. Caring for patients with cancer during the COVID-19 outbreak in Italy. *JAMA Oncol*. April 10, 2020.

into the exam room, after "foaming in" with hand sanitizer, she was sitting at the far wall, in a chair next to her daughter. Ordinarily we would have hugged, our customary greeting. Instead, I gave her what I have been calling my "corona wave"—placing my hands over my head, in a weak approximation of a crown, the virus's namesake for the crown-like projections that pierce its surface. She did the same. Whereas normally I gently grasp a person's shoulder as I listen to her lungs and heart with my stethoscope, both to hold her steady and to let her know 'I'm here for you, I'm on this cancer journey with you,' I didn't. She returned to the chair next to her daughter. I washed my hands again and sat eight feet away. We chatted a bit, even lingering, perhaps, so that our words, the eye contact that we made, our ability to laugh at each other's jokes, would compensate for the lack of physical contact. We sat in silence a while longer, the three of us.[156]

Hospice and palliative care, so critical for terminal cancer patients, also was jeopardized during the pandemic. An innovative telemedicine palliative care support unit was established at the Mount Sinai Hospital Medical Center.[157] Using palliative care physicians and medical students they developed a 24-7 help line for patients, their families and also to help support their healthcare providers, with smooth emergency department communication and transition.

---

[156] Michael A. Sekeres. Coronavirus and the cancer patient. *New York Times*. April 8, 2020.

[157] Ankuda CK, et al. A beacon for dark times: Palliative care support during the coronavirus pandemic. *NEJM*. May 12, 2020.

Dr. Shah, the oncologist who has experienced cancer personally noted, "The COVID-19 pandemic, although tragic and destructive, has brought the world together in many ways and made us all part of a bigger community where differences seem insignificant and we have a deeper appreciation of others. As oncologists, we are doing our best to protect our small cancer community from COVID-19 such that one demographic intersects the other minimally or, ideally, not at all. It is wonderful to see oncologists come together to build a registry on these patients with an intent to rapidly share these data to help guide management."[158]

Dr. Thomas Lee, the Editor-in-Chief of the *NEJM Catalyst Innovations in Care Delivery,* bemoaned, "I spend my day on calls and emails about Covid patients, and don't have much bandwidth left for patients without Covid-19. But, of course, they are out there. They feel like they are invisible—they actually apologize for disturbing us at this terrible time. And even though they don't have the virus, they are being deeply affected by the Covid-19 pandemic. Their care is changing—sometimes for the better, but sometimes not. From my own panel of patients and those of my friends, I could tell you about the patient with debilitating back pain for whom surgery has been put off until . . . who knows when? Or multiple patients with problems for whom emergency department or urgent care visits would ordinarily be recommended, but who are now deciding to hope for the best at home." [159]

---

[158] Shah, May 7, 2020.
[159] Lee T. Creating the new normal: The clinician response to Covid-19. *NEJM.* March 17, 2020.

The pandemic has reinforced the importance of integrated team-based primary care. I, as many of my colleagues, had been brought up with the traditional primary care provider, one fully able to care for me in sickness and in health. My primary care provider in Boston from 1995-2015 was in solo practice, working out of a cramped office at my hospital. He was the last physician on our large staff to incorporate electronic medical records in his practice. He was also the last doctor in the hospital to give up admitting his own patients and taking care of them in the hospital. The explosion of hospital docs, "hospitalists", essentially obliterated that time-honored role. When we moved to Portland, Oregon five years ago, I again chose a physician who works in a small private practice, independent of her hospital system.

Until very recently, I questioned the ever-expanding role of physician assistants (PA), clinical nurse specialists and other health care providers. I have always wanted to speak only with "my doctor", never really trusting other medical personnel in the same way. However, during the past decade it has been repeatedly demonstrated that interdisciplinary team management provides the best and most cost-effective care for a variety of chronic illnesses.[160] The clearest example has been in the care of diabetes, but team care has also proven ideal for the care of patients with chronic pain, hypertension and obesity.

Primary care is best delivered with an integrated, broad-based team of health care professionals, including medical assistants, nurse specialists,

---

[160] Wagner EH, et al Effective team-based primary care: observations from innovative practices. *BMC Fam Pract.* 2017;18:13.

pharmacists, behavioral therapists and IT specialists. Barnett and colleagues commented that as a result of the pandemic, "It is more important than ever for policy makers and government officials to increase investment in primary care. This increased investment could be used to help health care workers be nimble in how they will care for this onslaught of patients— deploying more community health workers, doing more population health outreach, and collaborating and building with their behavioral health colleagues to care for the mental health consequences of this pandemic."[161]

Dr. Daniel Horn notes that team care requires a different strategy, "Providing great care to a population is not about individual face-to-face encounters between a doctor and a patient—the way it is financed today—but is instead a team sport that requires expensive IT and groups of providers working together. What does holistic care look like during this pandemic? Perhaps the safest way to treat frail elders is to visit their homes. Contact tracers and community health workers may become a part of every patient's care team. Many more patients will need mental health and addiction treatment than we can currently serve. But the fee-for-service system doesn't allow for the sort of flexibility and adaptation required to meet these needs."[162] Dr. Horn and colleagues envisioned the ideal scenario, "You go to your primary care practice amid a bout of depression and are immediately able to see a behavioral health provider. You struggle with alcohol use or opioid addiction and a recovery coach checks in with you weekly as you pursue recovery. Your loved one

[161] Barnett ML, et al Covid-19 and the upcoming financial crisis in health care. *NEJM.* Apr 29, 2020.
[162] Horn D, *et al.*

develops dementia and a nurse case manager helps coordinate his or her care. If we change the way we pay for primary care, that's the kind of care our nation could attain. In the current system, though, almost none of these members of the health care team generate significant revenue, so most practices can't afford to hire them. Like airlines, primary care has long depended on people showing up. But unlike air travel, primary care's role of keeping people healthy continues—and is arguably even more important—when people stay home. The Covid-19 crisis is revealing the financial peril of relying on billable, in-person visits as the main way to pay for primary care, which provides little backstop in times of crisis. Let's heed the lesson of the Covid-19 crisis to protect primary care."[163]

Home care may become a more integral part of clinical practice. This may include "hospital-at-home" care, as well as post-hospitalization care. As detailed in a recent review published in *JAMA*, "As an example of how hospital-at-home care could work, a patient with congestive heart failure presenting to an emergency department would receive an initial evaluation including imaging and blood tests. If the patient required hospitalization, the emergency department staff would consult with a hospitalist, who would determine whether the patient is appropriate for hospital-at-home care and coordinate their transfer home, including any necessary tests, drugs, or equipment. The patient would thereafter receive 24/7 nursing care through a combination of virtual and in-person visits and be seen each day by a doctor

---

[163] Ibid.

until they could be shifted back to self-care or care from a family member."[164] Some countries have set up a Covid-19 home hospitalization unit. Patients are provided with a set of instruments and apply them while video consulting with a health care professional. Temperature and pulse rate are taken and with a camera/video device, the throat and lungs can be examined.

Leaders at New York Presbyterian Hospital described the complexities of moving telemedicine forward at their institution, "For our physician practice offices, we will coordinate same-day patient visits across multiple providers and streamline diagnostic procedures (labs, imaging, and so on). We will use telemedicine as a first step to meet patient needs and register all patients before the visit or procedure. We will ensure appropriate spacing for patients depending on vulnerability, increase time between appointments, and provide free parking for all patients at all facilities. Overall, we will limit exposure to others in public areas (elevators, waiting rooms), provide prescreening stations upon entry, and staff will cover multiple roles in the practice setting where positions can be cross-trained in order to limit in-person interactions for patients. The transition is going to be challenging—in many ways more difficult than it was to "pause" for this crisis—because none of us will be returning to business as usual. We are all facing tremendous economic uncertainty. The trajectory of this disease and the patient's response to expanded health care services are unknown."[165]

---

[164] Nundy S, et al. Hospital-at-home to support COVID-19 surge-Time to bring down the walls? *JAMA* May 1, 2020.

[165] Forese LL, et al. Restarting with Covid-19: Seven Key Action Items *NEJM*. May 7, 2020.

Hospitals, extended care facilities and physician offices are already rethinking their facility and scheduling to isolate those with potential infection from the rest of the patients. It is likely that hospitals will continue to have separate floors, triage areas, respiratory units. Offices will have "well-visit" sessions apart from urgent visits. Specific nursing homes will be designated as capable of caring for residents with recent infection.

Some countries have been way ahead of the United States in refiguring their healthcare with impressive early results. For example, South Korea has had a low rate of infections in healthcare workers and low population death rate following a rapid reorganization of their health system.[166] They implemented triage and risk assessment for any potentially infected patient and were quickly able to separate suspected or confirmed but asymptomatic patients from those needing monitoring and from acutely ill patients. Dormitories and residential facilities were used for those patients requiring minimal medical care. Specific hospitals were designated to be COVID-19 care centers.

Technical innovations have advanced at-home testing for various chronic diseases. The care of diabetes has been revolutionized by implanted glucose self-monitoring. People with sleep disorders, including sleep apnea, can better manage those conditions using various apps. Digital cardiac monitoring has exploded. I, like 10 percent of older men, have atrial fibrillation. I self-check my blood pressure at home. My Apple Watch has an ECG app so I can check to see if I am in atrial fibrillation. Every 4 months my heart rhythm

---

[166] Kim J-H, et al. How South Korea responded to the Covid-19 outbreak in Daegu. *NEJM*. June 3, 2020.

and pacemaker check-ups are done at home and sent online to my cardiologist. If something goes wrong, I get an automatic alarm. The pulse oximeter that has been recommended for people with possible COVID-19 to monitor blood oxygen is being fashioned into a smartwatch.

Comments from clinicians and executives involved with these digital advances[167]:

- "People are rightfully cautious about visiting hospitals right now, so being able to get any readings from patients while they're in their home is an advantage."

- "The changes being made now have opened people's minds to how they can deploy technology in a way that was different from what they thought of, even when we get
back to a level of normalcy."

- "I'd wager that over the next few years virtually all the heart-monitoring technology will be patches, or an Apple Watch, for example."

The most ambitious pandemic-related digital device seeks to identify early warning signs of an infection. A wearable device can be programmed to detect increased body temperature, heart rate or other signs of potential infection. Investigators at the Scripps Clinic in California had already studied this device on 50,000 people with seasonal influenza. Dr. Eric Topol, director of the Scripps Research Translational Institute, predicted, "The sooner we can

[167] Erin Brodwin. Fueled by the Covid-19 pandemic, remote monitoring could become tech's next big target. *STAT*. May 13, 2020.

recruit and enroll a large number of people, the sooner we'll have a chance to predict an outbreak. This is an outbreak that's going to go on for 18 months in cycles, but right now is the one that's wreaking havoc. The sooner we can get on board the better, "We've got to get ahead of this outbreak. It's obviously gotten ahead of us."[168]

Dr. Thomas Lee asks the two questions that are most on the mind of clinicians as we move forward[169]: "Will things ever go back to the way they were? and Are there things we are doing now that will become part of the "new normal?" He forecasts, "The answer to the first question is almost surely no. The Covid-19 pandemic is going to be one of those dichotomous events that divides life into before and after. We live through them, learn from them, and adjust. The answer to the second question, for good reasons, is almost surely yes — and not just certain high-reliability practices for behaviors like hand hygiene. We are actively redesigning the way we deliver care to do what is best for our patients during this time of crisis. Some aspects of that redesign will likely persist after the crisis has passed."[170]

---

[168] Erin Brodwin. We're racing against the clock': Researchers test wearables as an early warning system for Covid-19. *STAT.* March 26, 2020.
[169] Lee T. 2020.
[170] *Ibid*

4
Mental Health Fallout, Chronic Suffering

In Patients Recovering from Acute COVID-19 Infection

Most people make a complete recovery after COVID-19 infection. However, a substantial number of individuals have experienced persistent symptoms. These symptoms usually include depression, anxiety, cognitive disturbances, sleep disturbances, exhaustion and chronic pain. There are several possible causes of these lingering health ailments.

Either from direct viral invasion or associated immune-mediated inflammation, the infection may cause chronic tissue damage. The most obvious example would be chronic lung disease following COVID pneumonia, more likely to occur in smokers or those with pre-existing lung disease. We know that the coronaviruses can enter the central nervous system, causing an encephalopathy, presenting as confusion, delirium, seizures, as well as the more common loss of taste and smell. In previous studies of SARS and MERS, as well as recent studies in COVID-19, there is evidence for viral tissue invasion and inflammation causing acute delirium and other neuropsychiatric symptoms. Usually such neurologic symptoms disappear after the acute illness abates.

Another possibility is that the infection depletes so much of a person's energy, it simply takes a long time to recover. Dr. Alessandro Venturi, the director of the San Matteo hospital in the Lombardy town of Pavia commented, "We have seen many cases in which people take a long, long time to recover. It's not the sickness that lasts for 60 days, it is the convalescence. It's a very long convalescence.[171]

Many of the chronic symptoms following COVID-19 infection are likely related to post-traumatic stress. This triggers mood, sleep, and cognitive disturbances as well as increased pain in many parts of the body. In survivors of critical illness, at one year, the prevalence of depression is 29 percent, anxiety 34 percent and post-traumatic stress disorder (PTSD) 34 percent and in SARS and MERS, post-traumatic stress symptoms were present in 15 percent of patients, lasting up to three years.[172] Dr. Annalisa Malara, an intensive care physician in Codogno, Italy, said there was still no clear understanding of why the virus and its effects lingered so long, "Lack of energy and the sensation of

---

[171] Jason Horowitz. Surviving Covid-19 may not feel like recovery for some. *New York Times*. May 10, 2020.

[172] Rogers JP, et al. Psychiatric and neuropsychiatric presentations associated with severe coronavirus infections: a systematic review and meta-analysis with comparison to the COVID-19 pandemic. *Lancet Psychiatry*. May 18, 2020.

broken bones even after the more intense symptoms are gone. But even some of the infected who have avoided pneumonia describe a maddeningly persistent and unpredictable illness, with unexpected symptoms. Bones feel broken. The senses dull. Stomachs are constantly upset. There are good days and then bad days without apparent rhyme nor reason. The afflicted find the simplest tasks taxing.[173]

Recent news coverage has described patients with such post-pandemic symptoms. Fiona Lowenstein, a writer and yoga teacher, explained her symptoms after being hospitalized for COVID infection, "It's been almost four weeks since I first became sick, and three weeks since I was discharged from the hospital. While my fever and severe shortness of breath have disappeared, my road to recovery has been far from linear. My second week of illness brought worsened GI issues, loss of smell, and intense sinus pressure. In the time since, I've experienced fatigue, intense headaches, continued congestion, a sore throat, trouble focusing and short-term memory loss. Even more confusing than the arrival of new symptoms is the way my progress seems to stop and start. While the overall trajectory has been one of improvement, good days are often followed by bad ones, and I'm still far from my normal, active self. Lowenstein joined a post-COVID patient support group where, "Almost all are experiencing mental health problems, including severe anxiety, panic attacks and depression, as they struggle to understand what's next for them. In

---

[173] *Ibid*

addition to the physical symptoms that still keep me up at night, I have frequent nightmares in which I am once again gasping for breath.[174]

Dr Daniela Lamas, a critical-care doctor, talked about the need for dedicated Covid-19 post-acute care facilities, "At least we know how to track and treat the physical consequences of our patients' prolonged I.C.U. stays. These outcomes are visible. More insidious are the potential psychiatric and cognitive dysfunction that some former I.C.U. patients describe—anxiety and depression; hyperarousal and flashbacks to delirium-induced hallucinations that are characteristic of post-traumatic stress; poor planning skills and forgetfulness that might make it hard to remember medications or appointments. These are far trickier to screen for and to treat. Of course, it is early still, and we do not yet know the burden of these outcomes in our Covid-19 survivors. But given their protracted critical-care stays and the persistent isolation that so many of them endure, these issues will be widespread."[175]

Dhruv Khullar wrote about the challenges of post-COVID-19 care in the April 23 issue of *The New Yorker*, "The joy we all feel when patients at our hospital survive acute covid-19 is followed, quickly, by the acknowledgment that it could be a long time before they fully recover, if they ever do. Many will suffer through months of rehabilitation in unfamiliar facilities, cared for by masked strangers, unable to receive friends or loved ones. Families who just weeks ago had been happy, healthy, and intact now face the prospect of prolonged separation. Many spouses and children will become caregivers,

---

[174] Fiona Lowenstein. We need to talk about what coronavirus recoveries look like." *The New York Times*. April 13, 2020.
[175] *Ibid*

92

which comes with its own emotional and physical challenges. Roughly two-thirds of family caregivers show depressive symptoms after a loved one's stay in the I.C.U. Many continue to struggle years later."[176]

Dr. Lindsay Lief, a critical-care physician, runs a clinic for patients with post-ICU syndrome, "We try to offer holistic, whole-person care. Sometimes patients have already seen twenty doctors. They've had their scars, lungs, and eyeballs examined, but no one has asked, 'How are you doing with all this?' Often, what these patients need is not a doctor. They need physical therapy, occupational therapy, social interaction, case managers, financial planners. They need people to help them get their lives back."[177] Dr Khullar is planning to create a similar, covid-19 survivors' unit.

Every major traumatic event brings an aftermath of these stress-related chronic symptoms. In times of war they have been labelled as battle fatigue or Gulf War syndrome. Often, an infectious agent has been incriminated when a cluster of cases with chronic fatigue and pain are first described. Examples have included chronic Epstein-Barr syndrome and chronic Lyme disease. In such instances the symptoms were not the result of persistent infection but rather a biopsychological response to chronic stress. This is already happening in patients who were infected and very likely spilling over to the general population.

---

[176] Dhruv Khullar. The challenges of post-COVID-19 care. *The New Yorker*. April 23, 2020.
[177] *Ibid*

In the Rest of Us

While the direct physical impact of COVID-19 is limited to those of us who become infected, the emotional impact will likely affect every one of us. During the early outbreaks in China, the prevalence of depression in the general population was 48 percent and anxiety was 23 percent.[178] More than 50 percent of 1200 residents from 200 cities in China rated the psychological impact of the pandemic as moderate or severe.[179] In an Italian study, 30 percent of the population had moderate to major depressive symptoms and 20 percent moderate to severe anxiety.[180] Most population studies during the past decade prior to the pandemic have found a prevalence of depression and/or anxiety around 10 percent. This suggests that mood disturbances are two to three times higher in the general population since the onset of the pandemic. Insomnia was three times higher than before the pandemic. In China, sleep disturbances have doubled in the general population since the pandemic began.[181] Sleep disturbances were reported in 70 percent of hospitalized COVID patients and 40-50 percent of their health care workers.[182]

---

[178] Gao J, et al. Mental health problems and social media exposure during COVID-19 outbreak. *PLoS ONE*. 2020. 15(4): e0231924.

[179] Wang C, et al. Immediate Psychological Responses and Associated Factors during the Initial Stage of the 2019 Coronavirus Disease (COVID-19) Epidemic among the General Population in China. *Int J Environ Res Public Health*. 2020 Mar 6;17(5).

[180] Mazza, et al. A Nationwide Survey of Psychological Distress among Italian People during the COVID-19 Pandemic: Immediate Psychological Responses and Associated Factors. *Int J Environ Res Public Health*. 2020, 17(9), 3165;

[181] Huang Y, et al. Generalized anxiety disorder, depressive symptoms and sleep quality during COVID-19 outbreak in China: a web-based cross-sectional survey. *Psychiatry Res*. 2020 Jun:288:112954.

[182] Lai J, et al. 2020.

Prescriptions for anti-anxiety medications in the United States increased by 34 percent and antidepressants by 19 percent during the first six weeks of the pandemic.[183] One recent survey found that since the pandemic began, one-third of Americans reported symptoms of major depression, including exhaustion, insomnia and hopelessness.[184] *The New York Times* writer Nancy Wartik described her symptoms, "For quite a while after it hit, life wasn't bad. I had a job, at least, and was buoyed by family togetherness, by connecting and reconnecting virtually with friends. By the sensation of living through history. By walks in the park, observing fellow New Yorkers trying to fortify themselves, like I was. The last few weeks have been much harder. We're holed up in Manhattan, the future a fog without end. The days bleed together. Why get up? Easier to work from bed, especially as I'm tired and sleep deprived. Why reaffirm connection when I can scroll internet memes? And family members, can't they take care of themselves? But these aren't ordinary days; rather the state of affairs is a veritable petri dish for brewing depressive symptoms (sadness, insomnia, irritability, exhaustion, under- or overeating, trouble concentrating). We're locked in, some of us alone or in very stressful conditions. Tens of millions have lost livelihoods, and many are grieving friends or family. Normal outlets for rejuvenation — gym workouts, vacations, church, office banter, drinks with friends — are often unavailable. We can't necessarily make routine health care appointments either." [185]

---

[183] Express Scripts Report. America's State of Mind. April 2020.
[184] Nancy Wartik. How to tell if it's more than just a bad mood. *New York Times*. May 21, 2020.
[185] *Ibid*

Sleep and cognitive disturbances also correlate strongly with mood disturbances and chronic pain.[186] The risk of depression and chronic pain are the same ones that increase COVID risk: older age, multiple co-morbidities, obesity, smoking and socioeconomic factors. Just as we are in the midst of epidemics of obesity and diabetes in the United States, chronic pain joins that list. Chronic pain affects one out of three Americans and is our leading cause of work-loss and disability. Structural abnormalities, such as osteoarthritis, may cause chronic pain but most often chronic pain can't be linked to defined anatomic or organ pathology. This is termed centralized pain and includes chronic headache, low back pain, facial, jaw and neck pain and fibromyalgia.

Every large-scale disaster, whether man-made, such as the World Trade Center attacks, or natural, such as Hurricane Katrina, has been followed by a wave of depression, panic and suicide.[187] The Well Being Trust has predicted that "deaths of despair", defined as avoidable deaths from drugs, alcohol and suicide, will rise significantly as a result of the pandemic.[188] They predicted 70,000 additional deaths of despair, warning that, "Deaths of despair have been on the rise for the last decade, and in the context of COVID-19, deaths of despair should be seen as the epidemic within the pandemic."

Andrew Solomon, a professor of medical clinical psychology at Columbia University Medical Center, described his own personal experience

---

[186] Koffel E. Sleep disturbances predicts less improvement in pain outcomes. *Pain Med.* 2019. Sep 14.

[187] Neria, et al. Post-traumatic stress disorder following disasters: a systematic review. *Psychol Med.* 2008;38:467-480.

[188] Petterson S, et al. Projected Deaths of Despair from COVID-19. Well Being Trust. Robert Graham Center.

with mood disturbances and COVID, "For nearly 30 years—most of my adult life—I have struggled with depression and anxiety. While I've never felt alone in such commonplace afflictions—the family secret everyone shares—I now find I have more fellow sufferers than I could have ever imagined. Within weeks, the familiar symptoms of mental illness have become universal reality. Nearly everyone I know has been thrust in varying degrees into grief, panic, hopelessness and paralyzing fear. If you say, 'I'm so terrified I can barely sleep,' people may reply, 'What sensible person isn't?' But that response can cause us to lose sight of the dangerous secondary crisis unfolding alongside the more obvious one: an escalation in both short-term and long-term clinical mental illness that may endure for decades after the pandemic recedes. When everyone else is experiencing depression and anxiety, real, clinical mental illness can get erased. The authorities keep saying that the coronavirus will pass like the flu for most people who contract it, but that it is more likely to be fatal for older people and those with physically compromising preconditions. The list of conditions should, however, include depression generated by fear, loneliness or grief. We should recognize that for a large proportion of people, medication is not an indulgence and touch is not a luxury. And that for many of us, the protocol of Clorox wipes and inadequate masks is nothing compared with the daily task of disinfecting one's own mind."[189]

The enormous stress from the COVID-19 pandemic includes broad categories of:

---

[189] Andrew Solomon. When the pandemic leaves us alone, anxious and depressed. *New York Times*. April 9, 2020.

- Medical uncertainty
- Economic uncertainty
- Social isolation
- Constant media attention

This disaster has been unlike any other, as detailed by David Ropeik, a consultant on risk management at the Harvard School of Public Health, "There's never been a time in modern human history when every person is seriously worried about the same thing at the same time. There's never before been a ubiquitous threat that can be so instantly broadcast to a world of 7.8 billion people. We're being inundated with a constant flow of scary information that overwhelms our ability to be dispassionate. The stress of Covid-19 is now acute, but if it persists long after April, which it likely will, it will take an enormous toll on world health."[190]

Sarah Maslin Nir witnessed the anxiety from the pandemic in her fellow New Yorkers, "But with the coronavirus pandemic grinding on, that angst has reached new heights. Many New Yorkers are cloistered in their homes, often jammed tight with family or roommates; others must report to work in a contaminated city. They are dealing with isolation and fear; some have lost their jobs. Others are sick or in grief. It can be overwhelming, even for the mental health professionals tasked with easing such problems."[191] Melissa Nesle, a psychotherapist in Chelsea said, "Never have I ever gone

---

[190] Jane Brody. *New York Times*. April 13, 2020.
[191] Sarah Maslin Nir. Therapists and Patients Find Common Ground: Virus-Fueled Anxiety. *New York Times*. May 3, 2020.

through a trauma at the same time as my clients. All I am hearing all day, hour after hour, is what I am experiencing also." Donna Demetri Friedman, the executive director of the Mosaic Mental Health in the Bronx said, "I do a lot of self-care so that I don't take on the intensity of what we see day to day. But with this, it's so pervasive, there's so much death, there is so much uncertainty, the helplessness can creep in, in ways that it typically doesn't."[192]

Suicide rates have been climbing in the United States for the past twenty years and have increased since the pandemic began.[193] Matthew Nock, psychology professor at Harvard said, "It's a natural experiment, in a way. There's not only an increase in anxiety, but the more important piece is social isolation. We've never had anything like this—and we know social isolation is related to suicide."[194] Dr Nock has been using smartphone data to monitor people at risk of suicide, "From before to after Covid-19, we're seeing increases in suicidal thinking, among adults, that are predicted by increases in feeling isolated."[195]

Increased rates of suicide may correlate with increased gun sales during the past few months. Since February 2020, gun sales in the United States skyrocketed to 2.5 million firearms sold in March.[196] This was an 85 percent increase from March of 2019. Increased gun ownership is associated with a

---

[192] Ibid.

[193] Reger MA, et al. Suicide mortality and coronavirus disease 2019-A perfect storm? *JAMA Psychiatry*. April 10, 2020.

[194] Benedict Carey. Is the pandemic sparking suicide? *New York Times*. May 19, 2020.

[195] Ibid.

[196] Mannix R, et al. Coronavirus Disease 2019 (COVID-19) and Firearms in the United States: Will an Epidemic of Suicide Follow? *Ann Intern Med*. April 22, 2020.

heightened risk for firearm-related suicide. Having a firearm in a home is associated with a 2- to 10-times greater risk for suicide than in a home without a firearm. Persons who purchase handguns have a 22-fold higher rate of suicide.

Healthcare workers not only are at increased risk of COVID infection, they are at great risk for depression and anxiety. More than 1200 healthcare workers in China were surveyed during the first week of February and found to have high levels of stress and anxiety.[197] Emotional strain, physical exhaustion, shortages of personal protective equipment and concerns about infecting family members were of the greatest concern.

The April 26 suicide of Dr Lorna Breen, director of the emergency department at New York-Presbyterian Hospital, was headline news. She had just gone back to work after recovering from her own COVID infection. Her father tearfully recalled, "She tried to do her job, and it killed her."[198] Doctors in the past have had a suicide rate more than twice that of the general population, for many reasons, "We tend to be perfectionists…And disease processes aren't always straightforward. When you're a high achiever and you're very driven and you can't do what you want to do, it can be very disheartening. Now introduce a novel, wantonly contagious virus into the already chaotic emergency room, a virus that behaves in dumbfounding and pitiless ways. It's your problem to solve. But you haven't the tools to fix it—

---

[197] Lai J, et al. Factors associated with mental health outcomes among health care workers exposed to coronavirus disease. *JAMA Network Open.* 2020;3(3):e203976.

[198] Watkins A, et al. Top E.R. Doctor Who Treated Virus Patients Dies by Suicide. *New York Times.* April 27, 2020.

shift after shift, day after day, at a scale of suffering you've never witnessed. For people who are action-oriented and hellbent on finding solutions, this is a recipe for existential disaster.[199]

Dr. Tara Bylsma, 30, a second-year internal medicine resident at Boston Medical Center, recounted dozens of her patients dying each day, "It's so fast and it just happens over and over and over. You get numb until you leave the building. It's a terrifying, solitary, dehumanizing death that these people go through, and it's going to leave wounds in our society for a long time. That's one of the hardest things for me."[200]

Children are at increased risk of mental illness during times of severe stress. A survey of 1784 children in the Hubei province of China during the pandemic and just when their schools closed found depression in 23 percent and anxiety in 19 percent.[201] Those rates were significantly higher than at baseline. Dr Nadine Burke Harris, pediatrician and California's surgeon general noted the perfect storm for heightened stress in children brought on by the pandemic, "Our natural response to scary things is biologically to release stress hormones…exposure to stressful events — which right now might include the absence of routines, a parent's job loss and economic hardship, or the

[199] Jennifer Senior. What One Doctor's Suicide Taught Us. *New York Times*. May 3, 2020.

[200] Deanna Pan. Young medical residents worry their lives are on the line as they treat coronavirus patients. *Boston Globe*. May 5, 2020.

[201] Radesky, J. Supporting children's mental health during COVID-19 school closures. *NEJM*. April 24, 2020.

serious illness or death of someone a child cares about—can leave children feeling traumatized."[202]

Suicide has a close connection with social isolation and lack of connection, obviously in play for all of us during this pandemic. Family and friends have been isolated from hospitalized or nursing home loved ones. We all need to find ways to reestablish those connections.

Teenagers, already known to be at increased risk of suicide, may be even more vulnerable during the pandemic. Kathi Valeii described her own teen's anguish, "On a day when my 17-year-old son can't seem to summon the strength to wake up, I worry he's coming down with the coronavirus or that he's slipped into a deep depression. None of these kids had any choice in their separation. There was no transitional period to allow them to adjust. They did not know at the time to invest their moments together with the weight and ritual of farewells."[203]

Patients with pre-existing mental illness, the elderly and any patient with substance abuse are at increased risk for depression and anxiety.[204] Hundreds of psychiatric patients were infected during the peak of the pandemic

[202] Stacey Steinberg. How to keep children's stress from turning into trauma. *New York Times*. May 7, 2020.

[203] Kathi Valeii. Watching the pandemic steal intimate moments from teenagers. *New York Times*. May 15, 2020.

[204] Pfefferbaum B, et al. Mental health and the Covid-19 pandemic. *NEJM*. April 13, 2020.

in China and there were enormous challenges faced by these patients and their providers.[205]

People with a history of substance abuse face more challenges during the pandemic. They are more likely to be homeless, to be smokers with lung disease and are often uninsured. The services and treatments available to them have been interrupted or halted altogether. The new policy of relaxing the prescription of medications during the pandemic may further complicate the ongoing opioid crisis in the United States.

There has been a severe shortage of mental health care long before the pandemic. Even in countries with advanced medical care, 50 percent of people needing mental health services lacked access to care, including 12 million in the United States.[206] Before the pandemic it was estimated that 20 percent of the US population needed mental health care yet only 0.1 percent of the population had any training to deliver that care.[207] With the expected increase in mental health needs of the general population there must be rapid shifts in who is able to deliver this care. An expanded mental health workforce should include less specialized workers, such as community mental health workers, educators and other non-licensed professionals.

The difficulty accessing mental health care during the pandemic has forced creative approaches, particularly using telemedicine. Medicare has

---

[205] Xiang Y-T, et al. Joint International Collaboration to Combat Mental Health Challenges During the Coronavirus Disease 2019 Pandemic. *JAMA Psychiatry*. April 10, 2020.

[206] Marques L, et al. Three steps to flatten the mental health need curve amid the COVID-19 pandemic. *Depression & Anxiety*. May 13, 2020.

[207] Ibid.

already expanded coverage of tele–mental health services to include mental health counseling and virtual visits with psychologists and social workers. Thus far, no one has stepped up with a specific telehealth plan for individuals with suicidal thoughts. Screening for depression and educational modules, including those for mindfulness and cognitive behavioral training, have been available for a number of years and have been refined during the pandemic. Specific recommendations, not necessarily requiring a mental health professional, include:[208]

- Screen for depression with standardized questions
- Provide stress coping advice, such as maintaining routines
- Limit media coverage of the pandemic
- Advise on how to connect with people

Even before the pandemic we knew that chronic loneliness increased the likelihood of early death by 26 percent .[209] Guy Winch, writing for the *Boston Globe*, worried, "We can see this mental health crisis coming, yet we lack both national and international programs to address it. Here in the United States, a substantial portion of the population will have acute mental health needs, though there are few programs or mechanisms with which to assist with the emotional challenges our exit from a global state of emergency will require."[210]

---

[208] Pfefferbaum B, et al. Mental health and the Covid-19 pandemic. *NEJM.* April 13, 2020.
[209] Guy Winch. Loneliness, anxiety, grief-dealing with the mental health impacts of the coronavirus. *Boston Globe.* April 21, 2020.
[210] Ibid.

Healthcare professionals have been forced to be more innovative and flexible with all of their patients. Dr Michael Kahn captured this beautifully, "And then the pandemic arrived. To paraphrase Samuel Johnson, the prospect of a viral surge in a fortnight concentrates the mind wonderfully. Clinical priorities become much clearer; and indeed the experience of a few weeks of remote appointments has shown how shared danger calls for the kind of professional elasticity that can otherwise take a long while to discover. I often begin meetings not only by asking how my patients are coping, but also by surveying the emotional and physical health of their family and friends. Patients in turn ask me if I'm healthy and how my family is doing, and I generally don't hesitate to answer."[211] Dr. Barbra Zuck Locker, a psychologist and psychoanalyst in New York, described her telepsychiatry practice as a result of the pandemic, "It's utterly different and exactly the same. We've been seeing a move toward remote sessions for years. We have a sense of having adapted to it already. Most treatment, after all, involves the careful budgeting of eye contact. Patients look away, they look down, and finally focus, at a moment of intensity—a climax."[212]

---

[211] Michael W. Kahn, MD. Pandemic and Persona. *NEJM.* May 6, 2020.

[212] Adam Gopnik. The new theatrics of remote therapy. *The New Yorker.* June 1, 2020.

5
Managing Our Health

Information: Tuning in and Tuning out

We are caught in an information Catch 22. It is imperative that we keep up with the rapidly changing pandemic healthcare information but important not to become obsessed and overwhelmed. Ninety percent of Americans are following COVID-19 news fairly or very closely, but two-thirds said they have seen news and information that seemed completely made up.[213] Antonio Guterres, the United Nations Secretary General, said we are in the midst of a "…dangerous outbreak of misinformation and the antidote to this pandemic of misinformation is fact-based news and analysis. It depends on media freedom and independent reporting".[214]

---

[213] Amy Mitchell, J Baxter Oliphant, Elisa Shearer. About seven-in-ten U.S. adults say they need to take breaks from COVID-19 news. *Pew Research Center*. April 29, 2020.

[214] Press freedom critical to countering COVID-19 'pandemic of misinformation': UN chief. *UN News*. May 4, 2020.

We get much of our medical information from the Internet. The Internet affords us real-time information but provides no filter to separate the wheat from the chaff. There are more than 70,000 websites offering heath advice, most of them purely commercial. A spokesperson for the US Department of Health and Human Services said, "Trying to get information from the Internet is like drinking from a firehose, and you don't even know what the source of the water is."[215] The misinformation on the Internet, especially via social media platforms, is spreading faster than the virus. Dr. Vish Viswanath, Professor of Health Communications at the Harvard T.H. Chan School of Public Health said, "The sheer volume of COVID-19 misinformation and disinformation online is 'crowding out' the accurate public health guidance, making our work a bit more difficult, People are hungry for information, hungry for certitude, and when there is a lack of consensus-oriented information and when everything is being contested in public, that creates confusion among people. When the president says disinfectants... or anti-malaria drugs are one way to treat COVID-19, and other people say, 'No, that's not the case,' the public is hard-pressed to start wondering, 'If the authorities cannot agree, cannot make up their minds, why should I trust anybody?'"[216] An on-line survey by the CDC found that one-third of respondents were engaging in high-risk use of household disinfectants,

---

[205] Mclellan, F. Like hunger, like thirst: Patients, journals and the Internet. *Lancet.* 1999;352:39.

[216] Christina Pazzanese. Battling the 'pandemic of misinformation.' *The Harvard Gazette.* May 8, 2020.

including using bleach on food products, applying household cleaning and disinfectant products to their skin and inhaling or ingesting cleaners and disinfectants. [217] The authors warned, "These practices pose a risk of severe tissue damage and corrosive injury and should be strictly avoided."

Active disinformation has been fueled by greedy hucksters and zealots putting their cause ahead of science. Instead of sticking to reliable sources, journalists often fall back on time-honored techniques of novelty and conflict to push their sales. Facebook, Twitter and YouTube have increased their efforts to track and remove COVID-related misinformation, but it has been a losing battle. Untruths about wearing a facemask have contributed to the widespread disregard to heed this important public health measure.

Seventy percent of Americans want scientific/public health leaders to provide COVID-related information compared to 14 percent wanting political leadership supplying that information.[218] The best way to make people follow public health guidelines is for our trusted physicians to support those policies. As a *JAMA* opinion piece suggested, "We need to fight 2 pandemics—that of COVID-19 and that of misinformation. As trusted sources of health information, health care professionals have an opportunity to address misinformation and promote public health during this pandemic. But they need strategies to address misinformation that will not further overburden their time and resources. Educating people about trusted sources of health information, amplifying support

---

[217] Gharpure R, et al. Knowledge and practices regarding safe household cleaning and disinfection for COVID-19 prevention-United States, May 2020. *MMWR*. CDC.

[218] McFadden SM, et al. Perceptions of the adult US population regarding the novel coronavirus outbreak. *PLoS One.* 2020. Apr 17.

for public health policies when appropriate, and focusing efforts on vulnerable patients are key steps that providers can take toward addressing misinformation."[219]   Not every health care professional has the expertise, time or interest to keep up on the constant stream of COVID-related information. That was my driving motivation to write this book and get it out to the public quickly. There are certain trusted sources of information that I have relied on heavily and I strongly recommend to you for the most reliable COVID-related information. *The New York Times, Boston* Globe and *Washington Post* have specific COVID-19 sections with daily updates. *The New Yorker* and *The Atlantic* have published thoughtful, in-depth articles about various aspects of the pandemic. The CDC and NIH have patient sites available to everyone, focusing on public health guidelines which are updated frequently. The *New England Journal of Medicine (NEJM)*, arguably the premier medical journal in the world, has used podcasts and published case reports to illustrate novel findings or important teaching points about COVID-19. The medical *Journal of the American Medical Association (JAMA)* has similar podcasts and COVID sections. These two prestigious medical journals have made all of their COVID medical articles free, not requiring the monthly or yearly subscription fees.

The COVID-19 pandemic has been fertile soil for widespread fraud. Scammers take advantage of fear, uncertainty, social isolation and urgency. Fake testing set-ups, unregistered disinfectants and sanitizers, faulty face masks and medical supplies marked up 700% have been seen everywhere.

---

[219] Earnshaw VA, et al. Educate, amplify, and focus to address COVID-19 misinformation. *JAMA*. April 17, 2020.

"Robocalls" have pitched a coronavirus hotline targeting Medicare beneficiaries with this pitch, "Because of the limited testing we are first taking Medicare members. Will the free at-home test be just for you or for you and your spouse?"[220] The Federal Trade Commission received more than 30,000 complaints of COVID-related scams from January through April May 1.[221]

C. Zachary Terwilliger, the US attorney for the Eastern District of Virginia warned, "We are seeing fraud across the board, everything from low-tech to very sophisticated schemes, …the pandemic just allows the fraudsters to have their buffet, as it were, to prey upon vulnerable people."[222] While hospitals and medical professional on the front line were running out of personal protective equipment (PPE), a company called "Solo Supplies" had compiled a stockpile to sell on the open market of 200,000 N95 masks and 600,000 pairs of surgical gloves. Craig Carpenito, the U.S. attorney for the District of New Jersey, said, "It's outrageous. If I was married to, or if I was a health care professional, I would be horrified right now that I can't get the simple equipment I need for protection. It's just about the most un-American thing that I have encountered in my life. People are out there looking to profit, despicably, from the greatest national crisis we have seen since World War II."[223] "In Southern California, agents arrested a 53-year-old, small-time actor for seeking investments in a nonexistent company that he claimed was just days

---

[220] Ann Carros. Bogus vaccines, fake testing sites. Virus frauds are flourishing. *New York Times*. April 17, 2020.
[221] *Ibid*
[222] Sharon LaFraniere, Chris Hamby. Another thing to fear out there: Coronavirus scammers. *New York Times*. April 5, 2020.
[223] *Ibid*

away from marketing pills that would ward off the virus and injections that would cure Covid-19. The authorities said his YouTube and Instagram videos, in which he displayed a syringe of clear liquid or nondescript white pills, had been viewed more than two million times."[224]

Dr. Jennings Ryan Stanley, a licensed doctor and owner of the Skinny Beach Medical Spa in San Diego, was charged with mail fraud for selling "'Covid-treatment packs" that included the prescription medications hydroxychloroquine and azithromycin, hailed as a "concierge medicine experience" at a price tag of $3,995 for a family of four.[225] The package included anti-anxiety and sleep medications, all claimed to be "preventative and curative", according to Dr. Staley. His lawyer used President Trump's untested claims about the efficacy of hydroxychloroquine in Dr. Staley's defense, "The same executive branch that has been touting these two medications for weeks has now turned around and criminally charged an Iraq veteran, Dr. Staley, no criminal record, for doing exactly the same thing that the administration's been doing this whole time.[226] Intravenous vitamin C drips and other products to "boost your immunity", always pushed on the Web, have become instant best-sellers. Fully 15 percent of Americans have heard about

---

[224] *Ibid*
[225] Aimee Ortiz. Doctor charged with fraud after U.S. says he sold treatment as '100 percent' cure for Covid-19. *New York Times*. April 17, 2020.
[226] *Ibid*

these bogus claims.[227] *The New York Times'* Brian X Chen provided a guide to what to watch out for with pandemic scams[228]:

a. Fake websites. Check the websites URL. A good source is CDC.gov.

b. Install a spam or Robocall blocker on your iPhone or browser.

c. For possible robocalls, hang up the phone and call back. Remove businesses from your address book.

d. To guard against fake emails and texts, check the sender. Don't click on hyperlinks.

e. Check your network security.

f. Keep work and business emails and texts separate.

More than 90% of adults trust medical information from their health care professionals, about one-half trust the news media and the majority don't trust politicians.[229] Yet endorsement for unproven and potentially dangerous products has been rampant and is massively increased when we hear it from high profile people. For example, Google searches for purchasing antimalarial drugs increased 2000-fold after President Trump and Elon Musk endorsed their use to the media.[230]

---

[227] Mitchell, et al. April 29, 2020.
[228] Brian X Chen. A guide to pandemic scams and what not to fall for. *The New York Times*. May 13, 2020.
[229] Montanaro D. Poll: Americans don't trust what they're hearing from Trump on Coronavirus. Published March 17, 2020. Accessed March 29, 2020.
[230] Liu M, et al. Internet searches for unproven COVID-19 therapies in the United States. *JAMA Intern Med*. April 29, 2020.

On May 17, Trump announced that he had been taking hydroxychloroquine for more than a week, and "All I can tell you is so far I seem to be okay."[231] This will surely foster more unsubstantiated healthcare claims for unproven remedies. Dr. Steve Nissen from the Cleveland Clinic worried, "My concern would be that the public not hear comments about the use of hydroxychloroquine and believe that taking this drug to prevent Covid-19 infection is without hazards. In fact, there are serious hazards.[232] Dr. Eric Topol from the Scripps Clinic cautioned, "I think it's a very bad idea to be taking hydroxychloroquine as a preventive medication. There are no data to support that, there's no evidence and in fact there is no compelling evidence to support its use at all at this point."[233] I have been using hydroxychloroquine for 40 years in the treatment of my patients with rheumatoid arthritis and systemic lupus erythematosus and am well aware of potential cardiac and eye toxicities. Dr. Topol points out that fatal heart arrhythmias can happen even in people with no pre-existing heart disease, "We can't predict that. In fact, it can happen in people who are healthy. It could happen in anyone."[234] There have been a few, small, randomized trials suggesting potential benefit from hydroxychloroquine in hospitalized COVID patients but the largest obser-vational study of 1446 patients from one a New York medical center found no

---

[231] Annie Karni, Katie Thomas. Trump says he's taking hydroxychloroquine, prompting warning from health experts. *New York Times*. May 18, 2020.
[232] *Ibid*
[233] *Ibid*
[234] *Ibid*

benefit.[235] Almost 60 percent of patients received the drug and the investigators concluded that on the basis of these findings, "Clinical guidance at our medical center has been updated to remove the suggestion that patients with Covid-19 be treated with hydroxychloroquine."[236]

How much news is too much? We can quickly become overloaded with the never-ending COVID information. A study in China found that social media exposure was a prominent risk factor for depression and anxiety in the general population during the first month of the outbreak. [237] About three-quarters of us said that they needed to take breaks from news about the pandemic.[238] Nearly one-half said that the news makes them feel worse emotionally. David Ropeik, author of "How Risky Is It, Really? Why Our Fears Don't Always Match the Facts" cautioned, "We're being inundated with a constant flow of scary information that overwhelms our ability to be dispassionate. Our brains are screaming to give the coronavirus more weight, challenging our ability to recognize that most people are actually at low risk."[239] I would recommend that you limit your "COVID newstime" to one hour in the morning, such as reading reputable newspapers and journals, and then one hour just before or after dinner. Too many of my friends are catching up with the latest pandemic news at bedtime rather than lulling themselves to sleep with a trashy novel.

---

[235] Geleris J, et al. Observational study of hydroxychloroquine in hospitalized patients with Covid-19. *NEJM*. May 7, 2020.

[236] *Ibid*

[237] Gao J, et al. *PLoS One*. 2020.

[238] Mitchell, et al. April 28, 2020.

[239] Jane Brody. *The New York Times*. April 14, 2020.

Coping, Lifestyle

Combating the stress that we all feel since the pandemic began is no easy task. Stress is a result of anything that overwhelms our capacity to cope, making us feel out of control. Jane Brody describes our collective worry, "We're staring down an alien virus our bodies have never before encountered and which we are currently unable to control. There is no vaccine yet available to prevent Covid-19 or drug proven effective to fight the illness, limiting our ability to protect ourselves. So we buy reams and reams of toilet paper because it's something we can do to give us a feeling of dominance over a force that threatens to overwhelm us. But while a certain amount of worrying can help motivate you to protect against possible exposure to the virus, compulsively reading or tuning in to the bad news about Covid-19 throughout the day is unlikely to enhance your emotional or physical well-being. There are important health reasons to tamp down excessive anxiety that can accompany this viral threat. We have a built-in physiological response to imminent danger called fight-or-flight. Hearts beat faster, blood pressure rises and breathing rate increases to help us escape the man-eating lion."[240]

The goal to combat this increased stress is to quiet the mind. Methods can include simple distraction, like listening to music, my personal go-to way. For the past thirty years, I have often attempted meditation but never stick with a formal practice. Yet, during the last few months, I often do try to clear my

---

[240] Jane Brody. Managing Coronavirus Fears. *New York Times*. April 13, 2020.

mind, the secret to meditation, even for brief time frames. I might lie down and do a body scan or while walking outside focus only on each small step. I would also recommend any formal stress-reduction technique. These include cognitive behavioral therapy (CBT) and mind-body stress reduction programs, all available online.[241]

Keeping a routine is helpful during times of stress. My persona is well-suited for COVID-enforced social isolation and repetitive activities. I am a bit obsessive, always adhering to my rigid, self-enforced work, exercise and sleep schedules. Jane Brody's description of a typical day in lockdown matched mine to a tee, "As with life before Covid, routines can help foster and maintain feelings of normalcy and fulfillment. My alarm still goes off at 5:30 every morning, giving me time to enjoy a cup of coffee, set up my breakfast, check the day's headlines, make the bed and do forty minutes of back exercises before I extract my dog, Max, from his crate and take him to off-leash time in the park (his life hasn't changed!)."[242] Only differences, my dog's name is Charlie and I do my back exercises after Charlie and I take our daily walk. I have also enjoyed wearing the same outfit, an old pair of sweatpants and a t-shirt, every day. And I am not the only one doing this, as Billy Baker told his *Boston Globe* readers, "Another long-overdue adaptation that I'm taking with me when this is over: sweatpants. I'll need to get some nice ones for nice occasions, of

---

[241] Carlbring P, et al. Internet-based vs. face-to-face cognitive behavior therapy for psychiatric and somatic disorders: an updated systematic review and meta-analysis. *Cogn Behav Ther*. 2018;47:1.

[242] Jane Brody. Jane Brody's guide to life in lockdown. *The New York Times*. May 4, 2020.

course, but I don't think I'm ever putting on regular pants again. The first thing I do each morning is pick my sweatpants off the floor next to my bed and the last thing I do each night is put them back. We are one."[243]

Too much routine and social isolation, of course, is bound to have adverse effects on our psychological well-being. Loneliness breeds unhappiness. Five years ago, my wife and I moved to Portland, Oregon to be near our three younger grandchildren. Each day with them always makes me feel alive, vibrant and connected. It has been almost three months since I have been able to hold them. I began to tear up after reading Dr. Wendy Harpham's *The New York Times* correspondence titled, "Aching for My Grandchildren", when she said, "I'm again throwing kisses from afar, only this time through a window to my young grandchildren. I peer out from my post to watch my grandchildren clamber up the front steps. I revel in their delight at the surprises inside. The giggles grow louder as, with sacks in hand, they search for me through the double-pane glass to show me their treasures. Even though they recognize the toys, they love them. My arms ache to hold them close and feel their breath on my face. And here I am, coping with this 21st-century pandemic by kissing grandchildren through glass. In 1993 I could never have imagined I'd be reading "Chicka Chicka Boom Boom" to my grandchildren over FaceTime."[244]

Isolation has forced us to seek new sources of social engagement. We have set aside specific times of the week for conference calls with our family

---

[243] Billy Baker. The coronavirus resolutions we think we'll keep (but won't). *The Boston Globe*. April 27, 2020.

[244] Dr. Wendy S Harpham. Aching for My Grandchildren in Isolation. *The New York Times*. April 30, 2020.

and with friends, using Facetime, Zoom or other digital technology. My wife and I have taken classes and joined discussion groups and book clubs online. I am taking Spanish lessons; my wife is taking French.

Fortunately, my wife's outgoing nature and recognition of the importance of social interaction forces me out of my pandemic cocoon. I hope some of the lessons I've learned about connecting with others will stay with me but I wonder if, as *Globe* writer Baker predicted, "My bluster has involved preposterous promises following the words 'When this is over,' but mostly it has exposed the gaps in some of my fundamentals. I could stand to be a better friend, always. But it isn't just my social life that I'm seeing through a new lens. I'm going to be like the best person ever when all of this is over. You don't even know. Pushing pause on life as we knew it has unlocked an ocean of notions — resolutions tethered to some imagined moment in the future when we get out of this jail."[245]

This pandemic makes us think about our own mortality and pushed my wife and I to finally get around to writing out our future plans. Only one out of three adults in the United States has completed an advanced healthcare directive.[246] Dr. Jessica Nutik Zitter, a palliative care and critical care doctor in California said, "Without Covid-19 breathing down our backs, most of us look the other way from death. Even those of advanced age or with serious illness. But we are suddenly receiving a communal bucket of water in the face. Having a plan in place, one that doesn't sugarcoat reality, is the best preparation for

---

[245] Baker. 2020.
[246] Dr Jessica Nutik Zitter. Covid or no Covid, It's important to plan. *New York Times*. April 16, 2020.

ensuring that you are treated as you would wish. It also provides needed clarity to your loved ones, as we all navigate this pandemic together."[247]

Hopefully the pandemic will push people to adopt healthier lifestyles. We have already examined the profound effect of obesity and diabetes. Smoking and vaping increase the risk of lung disease, the main killer in COVID-19 infection. There are no large studies to determine whether there is an increased risk in smokers, [248] but most pulmonary specialists warn that smoking likely increases the severity of lung involvement.[249]

Recognize that we are all going through something very difficult and we need to talk about it. Dr. Neil Greenberg, a psychiatrist at King's College in London, who studies how disasters affect mental health, said, "What you shouldn't do is just cross your fingers and hope. The nip-it-in-the-bud approach is absolutely what we should all be doing. Otherwise your mental health could spiral down."[250] Craig Sawchuk, a psychologist at the Mayo Clinic agreed, "It's not necessarily that we're overexaggerating. An unusual set of circumstances calls for an unusual way of responding and interpreting. We have to accept this is a really difficult, in some cases, a tragic situation. You're human and this takes a toll. Look at your mental and emotional health just like part of your health, like diabetes. There are things you can do to feel better when you're diabetic. This is important, too. When we look back at natural disasters

---

[247] *Ibid*

[248] Cai H. Sex difference and smoking predisposition in patients with COVID-19. *Lancet Respir Med* 2020. Apr.8:e20.

[249] Vardavas C, et al. COVID-19 and smoking: A systematic review of the evidence. *Tob Induc Dis*. 2020. March 20;18:20.

[250] Wartik. May 21, 2020.

or wartime, when really bad things happened on a grand scale, the majority of people didn't get stuck. They didn't end up with clinical anxiety or depression. Resiliency is our natural trajectory. It doesn't mean we're unscathed or that we bounce back to exactly where we were, pre-stressor. But we can get to a better place than we're at right at the moment."[251]

Children need to vent their COVID-related concerns. Dr. Madeline Levine, a psychologist in San Francisco, advises, "The way you help a kid is by managing the sad feelings, not by denying them, not by distracting them. I think it's really important to let kids be sad, just as I think it's important for adults to be able to tolerate their own sadness. How could you not be sad at this time in history."[252]

Sleep

Sleep disturbances have increased dramatically since the pandemic began. A variety of sleep problems have cropped up, including insomnia, hypersomnia or too much sleep, and increase in dream sleep and more vivid dreams. On a typical night, our sleep gets progressively deeper, which is reflected by brain wave activity as monitored by an electroencephalogram (EEG). Most dreaming occurs during a sleep phase with rapid eye movement (REM), characterized by erratic, fast alpha wave waves. In deep, or stage 4 sleep, there are slow, rhythmic brain wave patterns. Most REM sleep, when

---

[251] Ibid.
[252] Melinda Wenner Moyer. 4 ways to help if your kid is depressed. *New York Times*. June 2, 2020.

dreams occur, takes place toward the end of the night. Even brief periods of repetitive sleep interruption or sleep deprivation result in problems thinking and concentrating, as well as physical and mental exhaustion. This may vary as to when the sleep is being interrupted.

Dr. Sanford Auerbach, director of the Sleep Disorders Center at Boston Medical Center reflected on the impact of the pandemic on sleep, "It's a very stressful time for a lot of people. There's a lot to think about. It can be very anxiety-provoking. We're not doing the things that help us maintain sleep— like exercise. If you're now sleeping in, and you're not just waking up because the alarm clock goes off, the thought is that people may be having the opportunity to experience more REM sleep. They're more likely to have dreams or remember dreams they wouldn't have ordinarily…some react to this crisis by becoming depressed. So, they sleep even more."[253]

Dr. Deirdre Barrett, an assistant professor of psychology in the Department of Psychiatry at Harvard Medical School, has surveyed 2500 people, asking them to recall their dreams since the pandemic.[254] A common pattern of dreams was "literally about getting the virus—that's been a fairly common dream where the person is short of breath or spiking a fever. And I've just seen dozens and dozens and dozens of every kind of bug imaginable attacking the dreamer. I saw an awful lot of dreams that seemed to be sort of practicing mask wearing or social distancing. In about half of them, the

[253] Stefania Lugli. What's up with our dreams lately. Sleep researchers cite extraordinary coronavirus stress. *Boston Globe*. May 6, 2020.
[254] Lauren Daly. You're not the only one having vivid dreams in quarantine. *Boston Globe*. April 24, 2020.

dreamer would be out in public and realize they didn't have their mask and panic or realize they had gotten too close to someone. In the other half, they would be doing what they were supposed to, and other people would not have their masks on or be crowding in the dream or be coughing on the dreamer. [255]

Sleep quality and duration correlate with health and mortality. In a recent study of more than 52,000 adults, those averaging 7 to 8 hours of stable sleep nightly had a lower risk of cardiovascular events and lower mortality rate than those with less sleep, with people averaging less than 5 hours having the highest mortality risk.[256] Night-shift workers suffer from chronic sleep deprivation. The disruptions in normal sleep circadian rhythm has adverse effects on the immune system, potentially increasing the risk of COVID-19 infection.[257]

In order to achieve optimal sleep during stressful times, maintain a regular sleep schedule. Wake up at the same time and set your alarm if necessary. Don't try to sleep in to make up for lost time. Don't read or listen to media coverage in the evening. Turn the clockface around so you can't check it out during the wee hours of the morning. Limit any naps to not more than 30 minutes and not any after mid-day. Exercise regularly but not in the evening. Use relaxation techniques but try not to force your sleep.

---

[255] Ibid.

[256] Wang Y-H, et al. Association of longitudinal patterns of habitual sleep duration with risk of cardiovascular events and all-cause mortality. *JAMA Network Open*. May 22, 2020.

[257] Rodrigues da Silva, et al. Does the compromised sleep and circadian disruption of night and shiftworkers make them highly vulnerable to 2019 Coronavirus disease (COVID-19)? *Chronobiol Int* 2020. May 20;1.

Exercise

We all know that exercise promotes physical and mental well-being. Any form of movement as opposed to being sedentary wards off loneliness, unhappiness and guards against depression. A three-month controlled study tracked the effects of aerobic training on mood in sedentary young adults who were not complaining of depression or anxiety.[258] After three months, the exercise group had significantly lower scores for depression symptoms compared to the controls who did no regular exercise, "…the group that exercised had managed to bump down their already-low numbers. After three months of working out, their overall scores on the depression scale fell by about 35 percent, a significant difference from the control group, whose depression scores had barely budged. Hostility levels in the exercise group also plummeted. The mood improvements also lingered. Even after a month of inactivity, the former exercisers showed healthier scores for depression and hostility than the control group…".[259]

Each of the chronic diseases that increase the risk of morbidity and mortality from COVID-19, including obesity, diabetes and cardiovascular disease, are improved with exercise and worsen when we are sedentary.[260]

---

[258] McIntyre KM, et al. The effects of aerobic training on subclinical negative affect: A randomized controlled trial. *Health Psychol* 2020;39:255.

[259] Gretchen Reynolds. Feeling down? Anxious? Hostile? A 4-day-a-week exercise regimen may help. *New York Times.* April 8, 2020.

[260] Jimenez-Pavon D, et al. Physical exercise as therapy to fight against the mental and physical consequences of COVID-19: Special focus in older people. *Prog Cardiovasc Dis.* March 24, 2020.

Exercise is particularly important to ward off age-related frailty and mental decline. Physical inactivity is a risk factor for poor health that is comparable to obesity and smoking and is responsible for 10% of all-cause mortality in the United States.[261]

On average, most of us lose significant levels of physical fitness after 1-4 weeks of being sedentary. Just a few weeks of physical inactivity can result in muscle mass loss and cardiovascular abnormalities.[262] Fitbit, the manufacture of all those cool watches, tracked daily step counts for 300 million users during the week ending March 22. They found a 7 percent to 38 percent average reduction in daily step counts compared to the same week one-year earlier.[263]

How much you move matters. A recent study in *JAMA* followed nearly 5000 adults over age 40 in the United States who were given accelerometers, like wearing a Fitbit or an Apple device, to track the number of daily steps they took for one week.[264] Then the subjects were evaluated about ten years later to determine if the number of steps taken daily correlated with mortality. Indeed, it did. Those individuals taking 8000 steps per day had a 50 percent lower death

---

[261] Dohrn IM, et al. Replacing sedentary time with physical activity: a 15-year follow-up of mortality in a national cohort. *Clin Epidemiol*. 2018;10:179.

[262] Carter S, et al. Behavior and cardiovascular disease risk: mediating mechanisms. *Exercise and sport sciences reviews*. 2017;45:80.

[263] *FITBIT NEWS*. The impact of coronavirus on global activity. March 25, 2020.
[264] Saint-Maurice PF, et al. Association of daily step count and step intensity with mortality among US adults. *JAMA*. March 24, 2020.

rate compared to those taking 4000 steps per day. This was true for younger or older participants as well as for gender and ethnicity groupings.

Your exercise should include aerobic, resistance, and balance work. The most important is aerobic exercise, defined as any exercise that utilizes oxygen substantially more than at rest. The most common aerobic exercises are walking, jogging, cycling, and swimming. For many of us, including my dog Charlie and I, aerobic exercise has been limited to walking outside during the past few months.

April Bowling, a professor of public health and former competitive triathlete, has been pushing her dog in tow workouts even more than me, "We walk the dog about 20 times a day, alone and together, go hiking and running outside. We're outside, every day, rain or shine, cold or warm, but we stick to places that don't have a lot of other folks."[265] April and her husband have also made use of the many on-line exercise options, "I believe strongly in supporting local businesses — your local yoga studio is more than likely holding virtual classes. Same with local YMCAs and gyms."[266] The pandemic has spawned a huge array of online exercise options and it is likely that many classes will continue to be held virtually, well after the pandemic is over.

For years, until the pandemic, I would alternate walking, swimming or water exercises with indoor or outdoor cycling. It's good to mix it up. I have become a big proponent of water exercises. My patients, particularly those with chronic back, knee and hip problems, found exercising in the water to be a great

---

[265] Brion O'Connor. Need a way to exercise? Get out and walk the dog. *Boston Globe*. April 13, 2020.
[266] *Ibid*

way to maintain fitness and strength with minimal stress on their joints. As health clubs open up, swimming or water classes may prove more acceptable to people concerned with viral transmission while exercising with others nearby.

Jane Brody, writing in *The New York Times*, recounts the same pandemic enforced exercise limitations I have experienced, "I remain devoted to daily exercise for myself as well. Unable now to swim every morning at the Y, I alternate between a 45-minute walk and a bike ride before I shower, don casual-Friday clothes and have a full breakfast. With so few cars on the road, there's never been a safer time to cycle on New York streets if the local park is overcrowded with erratic walkers, runners and cyclists, many of whom spurn masks."[267]

Health benefits are best obtained by doing an aerobic exercise for 30 to 60 minutes at least three times weekly. A common goal is moderate-intensity exercise, measured by your heart rate pulsing at 60 to 70 percent of maximum. Maximum heart rate in beats per minute is estimated at 220 beats minus your age. So, if you are forty, your maximum heart rate would be 180, and ideally you would keep your heart rate between 100 and 125 beats per minute for optimal aerobic fitness training.

If you have not been doing much exercise and are unable to get outside, try some of these tricks recommended by exercise experts, "During a phone call walk around the room or up and down a hallway. When you watch tele-vision, get up during each commercial break and stroll from room to room. Or

---

[267] Brody. May 4, 2020.

if you have access to a stairwell, climb a flight or two of steps. It may be only two or three minutes of activity at a time, but it all counts and adds up. For resistance exercise, do wall squats, pressing your back against the wall. Simply stand upright a foot or so from a wall, legs shoulder distance apart. Press your back against the wall and slide down until your thighs are almost parallel with the ground. Hold this simulated sit as long as you can. If that means five seconds, fine. Cans of soup or fluid-filled water bottles provide sufficient resistance for arm curls. Grip those objects with your arms by your side, palms forward, and slowly bend your elbows to curl the can or bottle upward. Lower and repeat."[268]

Being sedentary, an increasingly common pandemic situation, especially in older people, must be avoided. Anything that can promote homebound physical activity, such as online classes, physical trackers and smartwatches, will be useful, even when social isolation is gone. If confined to home, walking for 2 or 3 minutes, every 30 minutes, is beneficial. Jogging in place, knee bends, burpees and more intense structured exercise, combining aerobic and strength training, are recommended to achieve optimal fitness.[269]

It's okay to start slowly as Alexandra Jacobs described with her pandemic 'jogging' ritual, "For what I have done daily since this whole calamity began cannot fairly be described as running. Even jogging is, in truth,

---

[268] Gretchen Reynolds. Older and stuck at home? Expert advice on fitness. *New York Times*. April 22, 2020.
[269] Schwendinger F, et al. Counteracting physical inactivity during the COVID-19 pandemic: Evidence-based recommendations for home-based exercise. *Int J Environ Pub Health*. June 1, 2020.

a bit of a stretch. My feet do leave the ground, and so according to any accredited referee I am jogging. Just very slowly."[270] And you don't have to go far, as Jane Hu found, "Circling the block-a phrase typically reserved for vehicles in search of a parking spot, now something done more on foot-has become a near ritualized activity both extremely basic and extremely fundamental to my days. Call it pedestrian, but it is a holding pattern that has held me throughout my shelter at home. When I wake up, I circle the block. When the dog needs to be let out, we circle the block. Everyone, it seems is doing it. When sheltering at home, your world may feel suddenly smaller. But if your block, like mine, has slowly become integrated into your sense of home, then circling it is one way to make the world feel slightly larger."[271]

[270] Alexandra Jacobs. The joy of jogging very, very slowly. *The New York Times*. May 18, 2020.
[271] Jane Hu. The joy of circling the block. *The New York Times*. May 18, 2020.

Concluding Remarks

Since the focus of this book was to review the many changes that the COVID-19 pandemic has already brought about, I have steered away from much speculation on what the future holds. I have not discussed such vital issues as the medications being tried for COVID treatment and the promise of a vaccine. I have focused on those themes that reflect enduring healthcare transformations as a result of this pandemic.

We need more and better testing.

Dr. Vivek Murthy, Obama's surgeon general said, "the truth is, we are at best only 10 percent of the way there. Simply put, we are behind. Speed is everything. Time lost equals lives lost. It is your ability to find an infected person through testing—and then all their contacts—that matters most."[272] Epidemiologist Gabriel Leung of the University of Hong Kong told a New York Academy of Sciences, "This pandemic is not going to settle down until there is sufficient population immunity and the world is far from that level of

---

[272] Thomas L. Friedman. Make America immune again. *New York Times*. May 5, 2020.

immunity…until then this virus is going to keep finding people. It's going to keep spreading through the population."[273] Finding mild or asymptomatic cases and performing contact tracing is essential.

The pandemic has forced us to reexamine our healthcare delivery system.

Small practices are under great financial pressure. Shuttered hospitals and physician offices may no longer be able to provide care well after the peak of the pandemic. While our practices and hospitals redesign themselves, the public needs to again feel comfortable seeking any urgent and routine medical care. The handling of the pandemic in countries such as South Korea suggests that greater effort must be made nationally to consolidate hospital resources and systems.[274] Dr. Keith Corl, who practices both emergency and critical care medicine at the Warren Alpert Medical School of Brown University, said, "But patients and clinicians must ask, Is this is the health care we want? The cataclysm of Covid-19 offers an opportunity to reshape health care in ways that may not have seemed possible just a few months ago. Will we have the collective will to make public health, social justice, equity, workplace safety and the practice of medicine greater priorities than financial success?"[275]

Telemedicine is here to stay.

---

[273] Sharon Begley. Three potential futures for Covid-19: recurring small outbreaks, a monster wave, or a persistent crisis. *STAT*. May 1, 2020.

[274] Kim J-H, et al. *NEJM*. June 3, 2020.

[275] Keith Corl. When the Covid-19 pandemic is over, health care must not return to business as usual. *STAT*. April 23, 2020.

Dr. Donald Berwick, Director of the Institute for HealthCare Improvement, noted that "COVID-19 has unmasked many clinical visits as unnecessary and likely unwise. Telemedicine has surged; social proximity seems possible without physical proximity. Progress over the past 2 decades has been painfully slow toward regularizing virtual care, self-care at home, and other web-based assets in payment, regulation, and training. The virus has changed that in weeks. Will the lesson persist in the new normal that the office visit, for many traditional purposes, has become a dinosaur, and that routes to high-quality help, advice, and care, at lower cost and greater speed, are potentially many? Virtual care at scale would release face-to-face time in clinical practice to be used for the patients who truly benefit from it."[276]

The pandemic has forced us to be more aware of high-risk groups and healthcare inequity.

Our national epidemics of obesity, diabetes, depression and chronic pain have collided with the pandemic. More resources and awareness must be directed to slowing-down these chronic health forces. Hard-hit nursing homes and homeless shelters have brought attention to these vulnerable populations. Our racial and socioeconomic healthcare disparities have been laid bare by the pandemic. Minorities, especially African Americans, have been infected and dying at rates far higher than in the general U.S. population. As Dr Mandy Cohen, secretary of the North Carolina Department of Health and Human Services, said, "This current crisis lays out what we have known for a long

---

[276] Donald M Berwick. Choices for the "New Normal." *JAMA*. May 4, 2020.

time, which is that your ZIP code is often a determinant of your health out-come."[277] Berwick asks the big questions that the pandemic has placed upon all of us, "Is this the time for equity, when the evidence of global interconn-ectedness and the vulnerabilities of marginalized people will catalyze at last the fair and compassionate redistribution of wealth, security, and opportunity from the few and fortunate to the rest? This virus awaits an answer. So will the next one."[278]

We need to embrace public health.

Berwick reminds us that "No one can say with certainty what the consequences of this pandemic will be in 6 months, let alone 6 years or 60. Some 'new normal' may emerge, in which novel systems and assumptions will replace many others long taken for granted. But at this early stage, it is more honest to frame the new, post–COVID-19 normal not as predictions, but as a series of choices. The most consequential question in the new normal for the future of US and global health is this: Will leaders and the public now at last commit to a firm, generous, and durable social and economic safety net? That would accomplish more for human health and well-being than any vaccine or miracle drug ever can."[279] Antonio Guterres, Secretary General of the U.N. declared that, "Addressing climate change and Covid-19 simultaneously and

---

[277] John Eligon, Audra D.S. Burch, Dionne Searcey, Richard A. Oppel Jr. Black Americans face alarming rates of coronavirus infection in some states. *New York Times.* April 7, 2020.

[278] Berwick. 2020.

[279] *Ibid*

at enough scale requires a response stronger than any seen before to safeguard lives and livelihoods. A recovery from the coronavirus crisis must not take us just back to where we were last summer. It is an opportunity to build more sustainable and inclusive economies and societies — a more resilient and prosperous world.[280]

Albert Camus, in his 1947 book *The Plague*, a fictional outbreak of bubonic plague in Oran, Algeria, reminds us that "Everybody knows that pestilences have a way of recurring in the world; yet somehow we find it hard to believe in ones that crash down on our heads from a blue sky. There have been as many plagues as wars in history; yet always plagues and wars take people equally by surprise." Camus later in the book recounted what the world is going through now and his advice on how we will persevere, "There was no question of not taking precautions or failing to comply with the orders wisely promulgated for the public weal in the disorders of a pestilence. Nor should we listen to certain moralists who told us to sink on our knees and give up the struggle. No, we should go forward, groping our way through the darkness, stumbling perhaps at times, and try to do what good lay in our power."

---

[280] António Guterres. Address from Secretary General of the UN. *New York Times*. April 28, 2020.

Glossary

Azithromycin: A broad-spectrum antibiotic used in some early reports of treatment for COVID-19 infection, without evidence for any efficacy.

BMI: Body mass index, defined as the body mass, weight in kilograms, divided by the square of the body height, in meters, and expressed in kg/m^2.

Centers for Disease Control (CDC): United States Centers for Disease Control and Prevention, located in Atlanta, GA.

Chronic Lyme disease: A controversial term used in conjunction with people who may have had Lyme disease but continue to have non-specific symptoms, likely unrelated to Lyme infection.

Cognitive behavioral therapy: Any talk, discussion therapy aimed at modifying unhealthy health behavior.

Co-morbidity: Two or more medical conditions at the same time.

Corticosteroids: Anti-inflammatory and immunosuppressive drugs that include prednisone and related medications.

COVID-19: Also referred to as SARS-CoV-2 and Covid-19, is the virus, in the family of coronaviruses, that has caused the current pandemic.

Cytokines: Inflammatory chemicals released from various organs during inflammation.

Electroencephalogram (EEG): Test to measure various brain wave phases and activity and used to monitor sleep.

Encephalopathy: Diffuse brain inflammation as a result of infection, inflammation.

Epstein-Barr syndrome: Initially thought to be a specific, chronic illness that followed infection with the Epstein-Barr virus, subsequently labelled as chronic fatigue syndrome when no evidence of viral infection was found.

False negative: A test is read as negative when it is actually positive.

False positive: Any test that reveals a spurious positive result.

Fibromyalgia: A chronic pain disorder characterized by generalized muscle pain, fatigue and sleep disturbances, present in 3-5% of the general population.

Hydroxychloroquine (*plaquenil*): A medication used to treat malaria, as does its related drug, chloroquine, with anti-inflammatory and slight immune suppressive effects that has been used to treat rheumatic diseases, including rheumatoid arthritis and lupus.

Hypertension: General medical term for an elevated blood pressure.

Hypoxemic: Low oxygen saturation.

Immunity: Our body's response to infection or challenge to our normal regulatory mechanisms.

Kawasaki disease: An inflammatory/immune disease, primarily in children, that involves the skin, heart, lungs and kidneys.

MERS: Middle East Respiratory Syndrome, an epidemic from another coronavirus strain, causing sporadic outbreaks from 2012 to the present.

Mind-body stress reduction: Individual or group therapy that teaches stress-reduction techniques, such as meditation or other relaxation practices.

MRI: Magnetic resonance imaging, the imaging technique using magnetic energy to detect abnormalities in the brain and other organs, much more sensitive than X-rays.

National Institutes of Health (NIH): Agency of the United States government responsible for biomedical and public health research. Part of the Department of Health and Human Services.

Palliative care: Focuses on improving the quality of life in patients with life-threatening illness.

Pandemic: An infectious disease that has spread across the world.

PCR or RT-PCR test: Reverse transcription polymerase chain reaction: the genetic test used to detect active viral infection.

Pulse oximetry: Simple method to determine a person's oxygen saturation, normally 94-100% at sea level.

Rapid eye movement sleep (REM): Phase of sleep when dreams occur.

Rheumatoid arthritis: A systemic, immune/inflammatory disease affecting about 1% of the population.

Rheumatologist: Doctor specializing in the management of rheumatic diseases, including arthritis and connective tissue diseases.

Roth score: A technique to self-determine breathing adequacy calculated by counting to yourself while holding your breath.

SARS: Severe Acute Respiratory Syndrome, a coronavirus outbreak in 2002-2004, from different strain of the coronavirus.

Systemic lupus erythematosus (lupus): A systemic, immune/inflammatory disease often affecting the skin, joints, lungs and kidneys.

Telemedicine: Also called telehealth, includes any form of virtual, not face to face, healthcare.

WHO: World Health Organization: Agency of the United Nations responsible for coordinating international public health.

About Don L. Goldenberg, MD

Dr. Goldenberg was born in Milwaukee, Wisconsin and attended undergraduate and medical school at the University of Wisconsin. He completed his internship and residency at the Albert Einstein College of Medicine and rheumatology training at Boston University School of Medicine. He was Chief of Rheumatology at Madigan Army Medical Center from 1973-1975, then joined the rheumatology department at Boston University School of Medicine from 1975-1988, where he was named Professor of Medicine. He then became Chief of Rheumatology at Newton-Wellesley Hospital and Professor of Medicine at Tufts University School of Medicine from 1989 to 2016, Dr. Goldenberg is currently living on the west coast where he serves as a member of the Affiliate Faculty in the Departments of Medicine and Nursing at Oregon Health & Science University in Portland, Oregon. He is also Professor of Medicine, Emeritus, at Tufts University School of Medicine. He is an author and Section Editor for *Up to Date*.

The recipient of numerous medical accolades, Dr. Goldenberg was honored in 2008 with the prestigious Marian Ropes Lifetime Achievement Award recognizing excellence in arthritis care from the Massachusetts Chapter of the Arthritis Foundation and was selected as a Master of the American College of Rheumatology in 2009. Dr. Goldenberg has published more than 200 articles in scientific journals covering many areas of arthritis and rheumatology. He has also published 4 books. In addition, Dr. Goldenberg has been included in each edition of *The Best Doctors in America* and selected as one of the "Best Doctors in Boston" by *Boston Magazine*. His medical expertise has made him widely sought out for commentary on national and local television. He's been interviewed on the *Today* show and *Good Morning America* and his work on chronic illnesses has been covered in the *New York Times, The Boston Globe* and the *New Yorker*.

CPSIA information can be obtained
at www.ICGtesting.com
Printed in the USA
LVHW081526240720
661210LV00009B/51